Contours of the Flesh

Contours of the Flesh
The Semiotics of Pain

Darlene M. Juschka

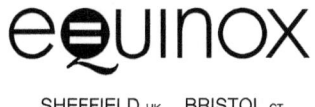

SHEFFIELD UK   BRISTOL CT

Published by Equinox Publishing Ltd.

UK: Office 415, The Workstation, 15 Paternoster Row, Sheffield, South Yorkshire S1 2BX

USA: ISD, 70 Enterprise Drive, Bristol, CT 06010

www.equinoxpub.com

First published 2021

© Darlene M. Juschka 2021

All rights reserved. No part of this publication may be reproduced or transmitted in any form or by any means, electronic or mechanical, including photocopying, recording or any information storage or retrieval system, without prior permission in writing from the publishers.

ISBN-13 978 1 84553 960 3 (hardback)
         978 1 84553 961 0 (paperback)
         978 1 80050 002 0 (ePDF)
         978 1 80050 037 2 (ePub)

A catalogue record for this book is available from the British Library.

Library of Congress Cataloging-in-Publication Data

Names: Juschka, Darlene M., 1957– author.
Title: Contours of the flesh : the semiotics of pain / Darlene M. Juschka.
Description: Bristol, CT : Equinox Publishing Ltd, 2021. | Includes bibliographical references and index. | Summary: "With discursive framing, this book works to make apparent the rhetorical play of pain demonstrating its social and political imperatives"—Provided by publisher.
Identifiers: LCCN 2020046544 (print) | LCCN 2020046545 (ebook) | ISBN 9781845539603 (hardback) | ISBN 9781845539610 (paperback) | ISBN 9781800500020 (epdf) | ISBN 9781800500372 (epub)
Subjects: LCSH: Pain. | Suffering—Moral and ethical aspects.
Classification: LCC BJ1409 .J87 2021 (print) | LCC BJ1409 (ebook) | DDC 128/.4—dc23
LC record available at https://lccn.loc.gov/2020046544
LC ebook record available at https://lccn.loc.gov/2020046545

Typeset by JS Typesetting Ltd, Porthcawl, Mid Glamorgan

Contents

	Acknowledgements	vi
	Introduction	1
1	Pain, the Body, and Signification	6
2	Mythic Caesura, Pain, and the Boundary between Non-human and Human Animals	29
3	Ancient Spartan Masculinities and Pain: A Case Study	67
4	Penetrating the Body of the Masculine Other: White Masculinity, War, and Ritualized Torture	106
5	Cut to the Bone: Pain, Foreskins, and Masculinities	124
	Afterword	154
	Notes	156
	References	167
	Index	181

Acknowledgements

This book was a long time in writing, as other projects and duties meant it had to occupy the back burner over the years. I am pleased it is done, and I want to thank my partner William Arnal for his thoughts and reflections on, and support of, the project since its conception. His insights were invaluable, while his support was a constant that allowed for the completion of the book. I also want to thank Kimberley Humphries for her editorial check-up of the manuscript—her assistance was greatly appreciated. Finally, I want to thank my loving children for their unwavering support in my endeavors, and their partners, cats, and dogs, along with my own cats, for the enrichment they have brought to my life!

Introduction

Bodies, Pain, and Signifying Systems

Many years ago when I was first on the job market I met two philosophers, one young and one older, where I was being interviewed for a position in religious studies. Throughout the interview and in my presentation I made it very clear that my theoretical orientation was feminist poststructural, and so at lunch the philosophers and I began a conversation. They held to an empiricist position wherein language, nouns in particular, images, communication, models, and so forth, did not construct existence, rather they captured and reflected said existence. Their position was that of philosophical realism; a view of the world I do not share. As we discussed our positions they presented again and again examples they felt made my rejection of philosophical realism untenable. But each time they put forward an example, a non-verbal two-year old fleeing in fear from a rattlesnake, I challenged the example. Why would the child flee, I asked, if there was not a communicative event? They argued that instinct, the fight/flight response, would take over. I argued back that for such an instinct to take hold, the child would have to *understand* that their life was in danger—that danger itself is an abstract concept and it is something we learn. Yes, the child could be startled by the rattling sound, but that is a very different thing from understanding the danger of a rattlesnake's bite. Unsurprisingly, I didn't get the job for a number of reasons, one of which was they remained as unconvinced by my argument as I by theirs. Such an encounter made apparent to me that those in opposition to poststructuralism continually draw upon what they think to be preverbal and anterior-verbal examples such as the prelinguistic period of children[1] or the human experience of pain, love, joy, and so forth. Indeed the preeminent scholar on pain, Elaine Scarry, has argued that "physical pain does not simply resist language but actively destroys it, bringing about an immediate reversion to a state anterior to language, to the sounds and cries a human being makes before language is learned" (Scarry 1985, 4). Following Thomas Sebeok (2001), among others, I contend that such "sounds and cries" are in themselves linguistic, part of language, and indeed shape our understanding of the concept and experience of pain in non-human and human animals. They are extra-discursive but this does not mean they are extra-linguistic. Judith Butler comments that "to 'refer' naively or directly to such an extra-discursive will always require the prior delimitation of the extra-discursive. And insofar as the extra-discursive is delimited, it is formed by the very discourse from which it seeks to free itself" (Butler 1993, 11). Cries of pain are distinct from cries of joy or sadness or hopeless, all of which are also linguistic and therefore part of our signifying systems.

When completing my text *Political Bodies/Body Politic: The Semiotics of Gender* (Juschka 2009), I realized my efforts to unseat the naturalization of gender and to demonstrate its ongoing construction through myth, ritual and sign-symbol would be useful toward challenging our epistemological understanding and certitude that pain (like other "bodily" events: hunger, thirst, confusion, age; or anticipatory states: pleasure and fear; or even those states of being named as "emotion"; love, hate, apprehension, and so forth) is not produced in and through language. To say pain is produced in and through language is not to say it is not in and of the body: the body and language are not separate, they are intertwined and co-constructive (Sebeok 1991).

Chapter 1 of this book is my effort to destabilize the thingness of pain and the body in pain, and to show how "pain" is socially and historically constructed, and therefore equally coded by gender, race, class, anthropocentrism, and geopolitical location. To do this I engage theories of the body, the intersection of the body with pain, and finally how the body and pain are played out in the representational narratives of myth, ritual, and sign-symbol. I engage these narratives as they are to my mind eminently central to "gaining the authority to bring about what it names" (Butler 1993, 13). Myth, ritual, and sign-symbol are "the conventions of authority" (ibid.) and not necessarily or only because of their content, but because they are some of the building blocks used to structure existence.

Thereafter I take up the body, all bodies, as sign and discursive and to do so I draw on the work of Jacques Lacan, Elizabeth Grosz, Michel Foucault, and Judith Butler, all of whom have influenced feminist poststructuralism, one of the primary lens that I use. The final part of the chapter brings Charles Sanders Pierce's semiotic theory to the body and pain with particular attention paid to the indexical sign and its delightful applicability to the problem of conceptualizing pain as a phenomenon and one that escapes language.

Chapter 2 is concerned with interrogating how kinship, speech and pain function to establish kinds of being and relations of being between non-human animals, human animals and deities in the texts of the *Iliad*, *Odyssey* and *Popol Vuh*. In the cosmogonic (creation of the cosmos), anthropogonic (creation of the human animal), zoogonic (creation of non-human animals) and demogonic (creation of the social group) myths, borders are drawn between non-human and human animals and deities by pain, speech and kinship as worlds are created. But even as non-human animals are set apart from human animals and deities, they are the means by which the ontological borders and pathways are drawn for human animals and their deities. The indexical sign of pain signifies strongly speaking to what it is humans, and their deities, think they can do to non-human animals.

Chapter 3 picks up a thread spun out in Chapter 2 concerning warrior masculinity, seen in the Homeric texts, and continuing to draw on ancient text, this chapter looks at how the indexical sign of pain is represented as central to the making of the properly masculine Spartan warrior. Seen in the film *300* and the graphic novel of the same name is a robust and indomitable Spartan masculinity that holds the tide against the effeminate and multitudinous Persians headed by the monstrous Xerxes, who threatened to overrun Greece. Occident against Orient, the film and the graphic novel (on which the film is based) created and glorified a white hypermasculine warrior, a warrior constructed in and through the indexical sign of pain.

Both the film and graphic novel construct a masculinity that is largely drawn from the writings of two ancient authors, Plutarch and Xenophon, both Greek and both enamored of Spartan masculinity and warriorhood. Both ancient authors provide narratives concerning Spartan masculinities and indeed both serve(d) as guides of ancient Sparta. In their narratives as well the indexical sign of pain plays a central role marking, as it does, the bodies of boys and youths. Deprived of all comfort and warmth, beaten and beating and driven to steal food, the boys are taught the hard ways of the Spartan warrior during their ritualized education in the *agoge*.

Rites and festivals expose and celebrate the pain the boys, youths, and young men endure and mete out shaping and reshaping the narratives of the Spartan warrior-citizen, who should give his life over to Sparta seeking, as was expected, a beautiful death. Removed from their homes during the Hyakinthia and placed in a mess, the boy engaged in ritualized agons wherein their mettle was tested publicly in the festivals of the Gymnopaedia, and the Karneia. How many boys and youth died as a result of these ritualized struggles is unclear, but not to enter the *agoge* and become a warrior meant one was marked as a trembler: the lowest and most derided members of Spartan society. Tremblers were given no wives, while their sisters and daughters remained unmarried. Tremblers lived with their shame of having been unable to conquer their fear and face pain and death, whether on the altar of Artemis-Ortheia or the battlefield. As Gorgo, remarks to her husband King Leonidas, when he and his 300 warriors were leaving for Thermopylae to battle the Persians: "Spartan, come back with your shield or on it!" This is a saying that was attributed by Plutarch to Spartan women (Mor. 241).

If the indexical sign of pain was a means by which to inscribe Spartan warrior masculinity on the bodies of young male initiates, it is equally the same sign that was used to signify the exposure of the inherent femininity of the Islamic other. Establishing hidden spaces within prisons called "dark sites," and developing and elaborating rites of torture, Chapter 4 seeks to expose how torture was ritualized and used at Abu Ghraib. In the US, prior to the destruction of the twin towers, torture was considered a barbaric practice and an anathema that marks the breakdown of social civility. Once the so-called war on terror was fully engaged, however, torture was publicly examined and embraced by the US government and its military. In order to convince US citizens of the validity of torture to secure important information, the narrative that torture could be professionally practiced and in such a way that sadism and loss of control were not aspects of the so-called proper torture was disseminated and performed. The idea of professional torture was, and remains, a fiction as Darius Rejali's work demonstrates:

> Some believe that all torture is the work of zealots and sadists, but studies of torturers point to the opposite conclusion. Organizations prefer to recruit ordinary people as torturers. Zealots and sadists are disciplinary problems, hard to control and manage. The problem is that professionals soon start behaving like zealots and sadists.
>
> (Rejali 2007, 455)

Regardless that torture has not secure good intelligent and regardless that the possibility of profession torture an illusion, torture continues to be used. Such use makes apparent there is more at stake that just securing so-called "intel." There is a need to break those others, those Islamic bodies, as a *quid pro quo* for the penetration of the twin towers of New York's World Trade Center on September 11, 2001.

Chapter 5 continues to examine the convergence and confluence of the indexical sign of pain and masculinities. This chapter is a genealogy of the cut to the penis tracing the indexical sign of pain in texts from the modern period to ancient Egypt in order to track the ritual cutting of the penis and the signification of the indexical sign of pain. Beginning with the WHO's project to cut the foreskin from the heads of black Africans as a means to stem the spread of female to male HIV transmission, the chapter engages five texts that speak to the cut of male circumcision using it to signify in multiple ways.

In this chapter, as with the others, it is apparent that the indexical sign of pain has much to signify providing insight into our and others' ontologies, epistemologies and metaphysics in the past, currently and in the future. The indexical sign of pain inscribed in the flesh of our being traces our existence as well as that of all life.

Chapter 1

Pain, the Body, and Signification

> I hurt myself today
> To see if I still feel
> I focus on the pain
> The only thing that's real.
>   (Nine Inch Nails, "Hurt")

Introduction

As a first step to think about the mythic narrative of pain escaping the parameters of language, this chapter examines the conceptualization of the body in feminisms of the late twentieth century and into the early twenty-first century. Since the body is the platform for pain, it is necessary to examine theories of the body rather than take the body as a given. The body, as I seek to show in this chapter, is a linguistic construct and as such so too is pain—both are signs within the vast semiotic systems that comprise our *Umwelt*. The concept developed by Jakob von Uexküll is translated as model and refers to the worlds that we construct in conjunction with the worlds we inhabit:

> Every organism is so equipped as to obtain a certain perception of the outerworld. Each species thus lives in its own unique sensory world, to which other species may be partially or totally blind … What an organism detects in its environment is always but a part of what is around. And this part differs according to the organism.
>   (Uexküll in Sebeok 1991, 54)

As Thomas A. Sebeok further explains, species see and interact in the world in ways that are shaped by the sensory capacity of each species although certainly these capacities must reasonably fit with its "model of reality" (1991, 54). For example a toad will starve to death while sitting on a mound of dead flies because these dead flies do not do what flies do—fly. The fly that does not fly cannot *be* a fly for the toad even if it is a fly for the scientist performing this experiment and those watching. The *Umwelt* of the toad requires that flies/food fly and not flying they fall out of the toad's *Umwelt*. As the world of the toad and human overlap in that both know living flies, they diverge when humans are able to see dead flies but toads cannot. Following Sebeok:

> Our intuition of reality is a consequence of a mutual interaction between the two: Jakob von Uexküll's private world of elementary sensations (*Merkzeichen*, "perceptual signs") coupled to their meaningful transforms into action impulses (*Wirkzeichen*, "operation signs"); and the phenomenal world (*Umwelt*), that is, the subjective world each animal models out of its "true" environment (*Natur*, "reality"), which reveals itself solely through signs.
>
> (Sebeok 1994, 11)

As part of the vast network of signs the body and pain provide ways by which we shape, understand and reshape ourselves and the world of signs we encounter every day. Drawing on the work of Judith Butler and Michel Foucault, Elizabeth Grosz and Jacques Lacan, this chapter engages conceptualizations of the body and settles on the feminist poststructural lens by which to engage bodies and pain. As central signs taken to attest existence, the body and pain emerge as core discourses to the discursive formation to subjectivity. Pain is the concrete index of consciousness, and reading pain and the body through the semiotic theory of Charles Sanders Pierce pain, the complexity of the signs of the body and pain are made apparent.

The Body: An Overview

In most endeavors of what is referred to as second wave feminism, the body is central to any and every analysis (and certainly this focus continues in third-wave feminism, but analysis began to taper off in the 2000s). This orientation toward embodiment is something that can be seen in the work of feminist theo(a)logians along with non-deity-oriented feminists working in the field of the study of religion. Outside of the study of religion significant feminist theorists such as Iris Marion Young (2005), Elizabeth Grosz (1994, 1995), Radhika Mohanram (1999), Luc Irigaray (1993), Judith Butler (1993), Susan Bordo (1993), bell hooks (1992), Susan Bordo and Allison Jagger (1989), Gayatri Spivak (1987), and Julia Kristeva (1982) have all contributed to feminist discourses of the body. Their interest and intersection with the body has been shaped in some measure by Michel Foucault's analysis of biopolitics (see Margaret McLaren 2002), highlights the materiality of the body, with a particular focus on its denigration and/or erasure in Eurowestern systems, particularly philosophy (ontology and epistemology especially), psychoanalysis, history, and science. They began with the female body (and then the intersexual body), since it represented embodiment in a way the male body did not, but then extended their work to ask about the embodiment of men (see Bordo 1999).

Inside the study of religion there have been a variety of texts, feminist-oriented and otherwise, anthropological, ritual, sociological and so forth, that have developed studies focusing on the body and systems of belief and practice ("religions"). Mary Douglas's *Purity and Danger* (1966) and *Natural Symbols* (1970) set the stage inside and out of religious studies for a sociological orientation; Rosemary Radford Ruether's *Women-Church* (1985) and *Gaia* (1992) brought a feminist theological engagement to the (largely untheorized) body; and Peter Brown in *The Body and Society* (1988) provided what was to become one of the preeminent sociological historical studies of the body in early Christianity. Susan Sered's anthropological engagement with systems of belief and practice dominated by women in *Priestess, Mother, Sacred Sister* (1994) made apparent the centrality of the body. Caroline Walker Bynum developed a phenomenological-historical study of the body in medieval Christianity in *Fragmentation and Redemption* (1991) while Naomi Goldenberg in her *Resurrecting the Body* (1993) shifted the analysis to bring together feminism and psychoanalysis since both narratives begin with, she argued, the body. Paula Cooey's *Religious Imagination and the Body* (1994) weaves her analysis through philosophical theology to speak of the body while Sarah Coakley's edited text *Religion and the Body* (1997) includes a number of different theorists, Bryan S. Turner, Talal Asad, and Wendy Doniger among them, who provide different approaches to the body, phenomenological, historical, philosophical, and sociological, with some few of these using a feminist lens such as Mary Midgley and Wendy Doniger.[1] These feminist thinkers bring to the table both a critique and corrective for the abjection and repression/rejection of the body in Eurowestern systems of belief and practice, particularly Christianities, as the latter have been hegemonic in the Eurowest for more than one thousand years, and around the globe with the emergence of colonization for at least five hundred years.

The discursive framing of the body follows several conceptual trajectories. Those who adhere to empiricism and philosophical realism take the body to be a natural object that is, like the real world, shaped by and in culture. The body as natural object is a reservoir for the subject, soul, nature, or a something that animates the flesh and bones bringing it to existence. This conceptualization is one that is central to the standardized model of the human, a model that is hegemonic in the Eurowest and certainly the one found in the majority of monotheistic systems of belief and practice like Judaism, Christianity, and Islam, as well as polytheistic systems such as Vodun, Santoría, Brahmanism, Daoism, Buddhism, among many others. In this model the body is a biological entity that exists in nature and nature exists in the world. In the Eurowestern orientation of this conceptualization of the body, humankind has separated itself off from nature, although in numerous racist and sexist versions those marked as "other"—through recourse to the body—are conceptually located closer to nature for numerous reasons (see also Ann McClintock 1995; Mary Daly 1978; Sherry Ortner 1974; Aihwa Ong 1995). In this version humans were once like non-human animals, but have over time acquired some aspect, reason, the soul, upright posture, brain-size, tool use, or language, which is understood to distinguish the human from non-human animal; indeed to remove the human from the category of animal and mark a sharp boundary between them. In this formulation those who have not fully acquired the necessary markers to qualify as "human" remain linked to the realm of the "animal" (Haraway 2003, 2008).

Another camp which also holds to the realness of nature and the body is represented by a feminist standpoint epistemology. In this orientation, the body is a natural object that is brought into social systems and consequently becomes a human being. Here, as with the empiricist orientation, the body is real biological entity, but this body ceases to be a natural object when brought into human social systems, and indeed from this material of nature the subject is constructed (see for example Harding 2004, 1998). This kind of understanding works to situate the body in time and space, and to make apparent that so-called biological norms such as skin pigmentation, genitals, callouses, sexuality, able-bodiedness, body hair, and so forth although real, have no *inherent* social meaning and only to *come* to mean, and therefore acquire value, in human social formations. This formulation of the body is often termed a constructivist position and the natural body acts as the ground for the construction of the "subject" in and through the process of socialization. In the socialization process we become "human" (that is a subject), and although those outside such processes (e.g., so-called feral children, infants/young children, sociopaths, the female/feminine, the racialized, and other others) are not explicitly understood as animals; instead, located outside the social they are conceptually situated as more in/of the natural world and therefore closer to non-human animals.

Feminist postmodernists, however, argue that the body is ever shifting and fragmented, acquiring meaning in and through culture, more specifically in and through language. In this narrative frame the body is not a fixed and stable thing in the world; rather, the materiality of existence *becomes* a body in and through human systems such as history, philosophy, language, science, medicine, systems of belief and practice and so forth. Central to this "becoming" of the body is language, for language takes what is not, insofar as it is unsaid and therefore unknown, and creates the body, e.g., immune or digestive *system*, flesh, bone, normal, abnormal, fat, thin, black, white, tall, short, etc. in the circumscription of "the body" (*le corps, quod corpus, el cuerpo*). And, even as it brings "the body" into meaning, that meaning is multiple and in flux shifting in time and space. In the postmodern frame "the body" is not singular and universal. It is instead plural and particular. There are *bodies* rather than "the body," and although there are similarities among human bodies (and with other non-human animals), there are also differences that cannot be erased or ignored. In this paradigm, the so-called natural body is a concept that operates within a binary system in the Eurowest (and elsewhere), a system that is valuative. In the binaries of body/soul and/or body/mind, for example, body is given negative value while soul and mind are both given positive value.[2] As feminists have aptly demonstrated, myself included, a gender ideology whereby the female/feminine is *less than* the male/masculine operates in tandem with the body/soul-mind binary linking the body with the female/feminine and the soul and the mind with the male/masculine. Various versions of this gender ideology were and are significant to legitimating and maintaining masculine hegemonies.

Linked closely to postmodernist understandings of the body is the body viewed through a poststructuralist lens. In this epistemological location, "the body" is an absent referent, being neither real in the sense of philosophical realism or biological certitude, nor neutral. From the outset "the body" is, to use Michel Foucault's phrase regarding sex, a dense transfer point of power (1978). The point that the body is not neutral I am certain most theorists would sign on to, but the body as absent referent is a little more contentious.

As I sit here typing with my hands, thinking with my brain, seeing with my eyes, hearing with my ears, my heart beating, lungs breathing, intestine digesting and blood moving through my arteries and veins, it seems rather nonsensical that I would argue that the body is an absent referent being neither "real" nor a biological fixity. I suspect this point requires some clarification. In poststructuralism and semiotics language is not merely, or only, a form of communication; it is more than this as language brings into existence that which we think we know and that which we are. Thomas Sebeok comments that "the derivation of language out of any animal communication systems is an exercise in total futility, because language did not evolve to subserve humanity's communicative exigencies. It evolved ... as an exceedingly sophisticated modelling device ... in *Homo habilis*" (1994, 136). Communication is certainly central to language, but it is not the only or even the primary aspect of language. Instead, language is first and foremost a modelling device or a way by which humans corporately and individually code existence and then subsequently decode and recode representations of existence already produced. Our worlds, or *Umwelts* (Sebeok 1994), are composed of signs. This coding, decoding and recoding of existence draws upon, as I have argued elsewhere (Juschka 2009), what Claude Lévi-Strauss has called bricolage to resignify existence. The process is *ad infinitum*—within the boundary of species existence of course.

Part of my understanding of the body, and therefore the human, is shaped by Jacques Lacan's (1968) psychoanalytic theory wherein he conjectures the orders of the Real, the Imaginary and the Symbolic with regard to human psyche-bodily development. Following Freud, Lacan argues that the infant is an undifferentiated being at one with all that is around it. There is an unconsciousness of being wherein the child has yet to identified themselves as separate from the (m)other. The child has no awareness of their corporeal boundaries, they are ubiquitous with no separation between themselves and objects since the child forms a primal unity with its objects. Elizabeth Grosz writes that:

> The Real cannot be experienced as such; it is capable of representation or conceptualization only through the reconstructive or inferential work of the imaginary and symbolic orders. Lacan himself refers to the Real as "the lack of lack." It is what is "unassimilable" (1977, 55) in representation, the "impossible" (167). Our distance from the Real is the measure of our socio-psychical development. The Real has no boundaries, borders, divisions, or oppositions; it is a continuum of "raw materials." The Real is not however the same as reality; reality is lived as and known through imaginary and symbolic representations.
>
> (Grosz 1990, 34)

Not until the infant enters the Imaginary order, initiated by the mirror stage (6–18 months), does the child differentiate themselves from the world around.

During the mirror stage the child (mis)recognizes themselves as a whole and separate from that which is around it, particularly the (m)other. In the mirror stage a split occurs and the child shifts into seeing themselves as subject and object (They who look into the mirror and they who return the look) and the order of the Real of Lacanian theory is pushed into the unconscious. The mirror stage, or the introduction of the Imaginary, refers to the act of self-recognition by the child and with this recognition the child is hurled into identificatory relations by this first lack or loss (loss of the Real). It is at this juncture that the child can distinguish themselves from the world and thus locate themselves *in* the world. Importantly, in the formation of imaginary relations with the world there is a formation of imaginary relations with the body and as the self is separate from the world, so too the self from the body: as the human is in the world, so too the self is in the body; as the world is outside, so too the body is the outside or external to the "self" inside (Lacan 2007, 6–48; see also Grosz 1994, 9–10).

The Imaginary is the order of identification with images and identification with images means a split in self (body and self). In order to recognize themselves as an image in the mirror they necessarily must become simultaneously an object and subject to themselves. The child recognizes themselves (body-outside) in the image but also recognizes recognizing themselves as an image (self-inside). The operation is dual and in the moment the image is recognized there is the knowledge of recognition and we are simultaneously both objects (the body) and subjects (the self). The entrance into the Imaginary is a loss of omnitude, and represents a profound tear or rupture with the Real, the latter of which then recedes into the unconscious. In the desire to fill the gap left in the wake of the rupture there is a seeking of an identificatory image, one that is stable and permanent (the imaginary), and eventually and entrance into language (the symbolic). As Lacan wrote:

> Thus, if man comes to think about the symbolic order, it is because he is first caught in it in his being. The illusion that he has formed this order through his consciousness stems from the fact that it is through the pathway of a specific gap in his imaginary relationship with his semblable that he has been able to enter into this order as a subject.
>
> (Lacan 2007, 40)

The final category of Lacan's new order is that of the Symbolic. The Symbolic is how we enter the social and therefore the means by which we are constituted as social entities: The symbolic constitutes the subject and their world (Lacan 2007, 7). The symbolic order constitutes our *Umwelt*, our "phenomenonal world ... the subjective world each animal models out of its 'true' environment (*Natur*, 'reality'), which reveals itself solely through signs" (Sebeok 1994, 144). The complexity of this category goes beyond this discussion, but suffice to say that language is both the law of the father and the rule of the phallus in masculine hegemonies. In order to enter language, according to Lacan, the dyadic structure of mother-child must give way to the plurality which constitutes the symbolic order. The narcissistic couple must be submitted to symbolic regulation, and because of men's absence and women's presence, the father, who is the third and breaks the dyad of mother-child, represents law, order, and authority to the child. However, it is not the real of the genetic father but the imaginary father who acts as an incarnation or delegate of the symbolic father (other authority figures such as teachers, policemen, or deity can also act in this role) (Lacan 2007, 149). Entering the Symbolic means a separation from the first love object, the (m)other, and a positioning within the larger social and symbolic environment of culture.[3]

The formation of the "human" that Lacan proposes I adopt but nuance particularly with regard to gender/sex, race, class, and other important identificatory categories that operate in the Imaginary and Symbolic orders. When thinking about "the body" in light of Lacan's work the body as "real" can only be an absent referent even as I sit here typing these words with my fingers reading them with my eyes and hearing the clicking of the computer keys. This is to say, the unrepresentable body that occupies the order of the Real is not accessible to any of us as it has receded into the unconscious and we exist as split selves comprising an object/subject, a body/mind-soul and an exterior/interior.[4] Kirsten Campbell comments that:

> Lacan posits the Real as excess, impossibility and lack ... It is the logical obstacle that cannot be represented within the symbolic (S17:143). For this reason, the Real is also lack in language, because it marks that which the Symbolic cannot symbolize. No signifying chain can represent it in its totality—hence its impossibility. Something always must fall out of discourse, hence its excluded *a*. In this way, the Real can also be understood as the hole in the Symbolic order, the impossibility on which that order is predicated and the absence that it encircles.
>
> (Campbell 2004, 131)

Lacan, was very much influenced by the work of Sigmund Freud. Following both Lacan and Freud, then, I adhere to the view that there are two systems—the conscious and unconscious (although I am less convinced of a preconscious), although my understanding of the unconscious is not particularly Freudian. Rather than a depository of repressions, anxieties and so forth, I take the unconscious to be the body and the body, which includes the brain, is that which communicates through somaethesis, gestures, whispers, rhythm, flashes, dreams, and so forth.[5] The unconscious was of great concern to Freud since it was central to his psychoanalytic practice and theory of the human psyche. Freud, like Lacan, links the unconscious with the body, although in the case of Freud an aspect of the link is problematic, shaped as it was by nineteenth-century thought on the body.[6] In Freud's theorizing, the drives were linked to the body acting as the border between the physical and the mental (Freud 2005, 632–642). Although the location of the drives in particular organs is nonviable, the idea that the body has a means by which "to speak" and to speak its knowing in and through the unconscious provides an agency to the body that is not often seen. Although Freud probably did not intend such a meaning, since in his work he was concerned with the psyche and for all intents and purposes this psyche was primarily located in the mind, his idea that the unconscious is a site for body talk is immensely useful. I will return to this point further on.

The poststructural proposition of the subject as situated, multiple, shifting, and unstable I also use to understand the body, as both the body and the subject are taken to be representations that are joined together to signify the human. The body—any and all bodies—as a thing in and of itself in existence belongs to the order of the Real and subsequently is unavailable to us. Judith Butler's theorizing of the body takes into account Lacan's three orders, while resisting the implications inherent to the constructivist positions.[7] She advocates the need to return to the notion of matter and to bring matter into conceptualization of the body:

> What I propose in place of these conceptions of construction is a return to the notion of matter, not as site or surface, but as *a process of materialization that stabilizes over time to produce the effect of boundary, fixity, and surface we call matter.*
> (Butler 1993, 9, emphasis original)

In this formulation the body and subjectivity are not separate so that one presupposes an interior "self" (subjectivity) operating and shaping an exterior and passive flesh; rather flesh and subjectivity are one and the same so that, for example, the individuation and separation of body and subjectivity, or body and mind, or body and soul, are not the truth of "the body"; rather they are the ideological effects produced in the stabilization of subjectivity and in this the body. And these ideological effects operative in the process of materialization are produced in and through discourse. Following Chris Weedon, then:

> the fundamental poststructuralist idea that discourses produce meaning and subjectivity, rather than reflecting them, makes language and subjectivity ongoing sites of political struggle ... discourse is more than linguistic meaning. It is material in the sense that it is located in institutions and practices which define difference and shape the material world, including bodies.
> (Weedon 1999, 102–103)

The poststructuralist refusal to define and fix the body means that the body is, as Michel Foucault argued, a site for the deployment of ideology (and resistance to this deployment). Naming the force that shapes and controls the body as biopower, Foucault (1978) suggested that there are two kinds of power asserted, disciplinary and regulatory. Disciplinary power is that which establishes the knowledge of and power over the individual body and its capacities, gestures, movements, location and behaviors; while regulatory power is that which is inscribed in policies and interventions that govern the population. Regulatory power is, he argued, focused on the "species body" or the body that serves as the basis of biological processes affecting birth, death, the level of health and longevity. Regulatory power is accomplished by state intervention through such instruments as demographics, public health agencies, health economics and so forth. Foucault argued that Eurowestern biopower emerged in concrete terms at the beginning of the seventeenth century, whereupon it was delineated in its two forms of disciplinary and regulatory powers (ibid., 145–146). The body, individual and species, unfixed and fluid,[8] is, then, a primary site of struggle and should not be taken as a given.

Discourses of Pain and the Body

The "body is a process of materialization," following Butler and drawing on Lacan, while this process of materialization begins in the order of the Real, moves through the Imaginary wherein there is a misrecognition of the body/self as whole and hermetically sealed, and then into the order of the Symbolic wherein the body/self is continually shaped and reshaped; inscribed as it is with those bodily markers considered significant whatever they might be, for example, human versus non-human, gender/sex, race, class, age, and so forth.

In the absence of the Real, which Lacan proposes, there is the manufacturing of the Real since this absence can only be "lack" and lack cannot be abided within the Symbolic. It is in the Imaginary order when wholeness is proposed that a manufactured Real—the body that is an animal body and is akin to the non-human animal, "nature," biology, for example—emerges. The manufactured Real thus becomes the ground on which all else is built even while it is shaped and reshaped in and by the Symbolic order. A product of the Imaginary order, the manufactured Real is a reflection of the Imaginary and Symbolic orders even as it appears to be outside of them. The Real is projected as primordial in both time and space and so too anything associated with the body such as pain, gender/sex, race, sexuality, or desire.

The idea of a manufactured Real allows for the conceptualization of the body as fluid and in constant flux, and therefore more along the lines of Butler's "process of materialization." In this formulation there can be "no reference to a pure body which is not at the same time a further formation of that body" (Butler 1993, 10). The body proposed to be real is (continually) constructed by and within the Imaginary and Symbolic orders and therefore is susceptible to the vicissitudes of time and place. In other words, the constructed nature of the body means that it is neither pristine nor primordial, a thing of nature, as it is commonly represented in the Eurowest.

If the body is constructed, then so too is pain. To say that pain, like the body, is constructed does not mean that pain and the body are not experienced. They *are* experienced, but that experience is equally subject to social construction. Joan W. Scott has convincingly argued:

> "[E]xperience" whether conceived as internal or external, subjective or objective, establishes the prior existence of individuals. When it is defined as internal, it is an expression of an individual's being or consciousness, when external it is the material upon which consciousness then acts. Talking about experience in these ways leads us to take the existence of individuals for granted (experience is something people have) rather than to ask how conceptions of selves (of subjects and their identities) are produced. It operates within an ideological construction that not only makes individuals the starting point of knowledge, but that also naturalizes categories such as man, woman, black, white, heterosexual, or homosexual by treating them as given characteristics of individuals.
>
> (Scott 1992, 27)

We face construction coming and going, but such construction or composition must be understood as fluid and on-going rather than fixed and once and for all. The body, like the pain, is constituted and performative and in the performance is reconstituted. Judith Butler points out that "performativity is thus not a singular "act," for it is always a reiteration of a norm or a set of norms, and to the extent it acquires an act-like status in the present, it conceals or dissimulates the conventions of which it is a repetition" (Butler 1993, 12). To say that the body and pain are constructed and performed is of course contentious, but not so if understood within a poststructural theoretical frame. In poststructuralism there is no effort to separate the false from the true, only the recognition that with construction comes deconstruction allowing theorists to investigate the body and pain as concepts since they "are no longer reified as 'referents,' and ... stand a chance of being opened up ..." (ibid., 29).

If the body and pain are constructed and performed, this does not mean they are not experienced. Certainly we experience the body and in, through and related to the body we experience pain. However, I argue here that the experience of pain is formed and mapped through a discursive framing of pain. In my experience of pain, pain invaded and took up lodging in my body, and my effort, then, was to manipulate (e.g., medical treatment, medicine, meditation, breathing exercises, knowledge) my body in order to vanquish or at the very least mitigate the pain. The understanding of pain—as that which comes to inhabit the body—locates pain outside and as something that overtakes one: "Damn I wish this pain would go away." It is not necessarily that one believes pain is an actual thing in the world, but it is an aspect of the discourse of pain in the Eurowest, if not elsewhere.

There are numerous ways that pain is spoken, a discursive formation of pain, as narratives of it are developed, shaped, and altered according to time and place. Pain can be figured as that which purifies (e.g., Glucklich 2001), as a guarantor of truth, (e.g., DuBois 1991; Silverman 2001), as a necessary step into adulthood (e.g., Herdt 1994), as a marker of courage and fortitude and as a marker of weakness (e.g., Burstyn 1999), as a calling (e.g., Danforth 1989) and so forth. The narratives of pain are legion. Sarah Coakley and Kay Kaufman Shelemay's edited text *Pain and its Transformations: The Interface of Biology and Culture* (2007) provides a collection of articles engaging the concept of pain. In Coakley's introduction she asks some very interesting questions about the discourse of pain:

> What *is* pain exactly? What is its relation to "suffering"? How many sorts of pain are there? And can physical pain finally be separated from what is colloquially called "mental" or spiritual" pain? Or are these latter categories theoretical mistakes? Further, is pain essentially private and incommunicable, reducing us to inarticulacy, to loss of speech (Scarry 1985)? Or does it provide the axis for a potent means of communication—a bridge to empathy and a deeper recognition of the "other" in the face of suffering? (Levinas 1969; Kleinman, Das and Lock 1997).
>
> (Coakley 2007, 3)

If pain is discourse it cannot be treated phenomenologically, as is done by Coakley and the majority of the contributors of the text. However, where our interests segue is in conceptualizing pain as a "potent means of communication." In the semiotic frame, language is a system of signs that includes all forms of representation including art, film, text, music, architecture, gesture, movement, drama, ritual, myth, icon, and sign-symbol. As Stuart Hall puts it:

> Language is able to do this because it operates as a *representational system*. In language we use signs and symbols—whether they are sounds, written words, electronically produced images, musical notes, even objects—to stand for or represent to other people our concepts, ideas and feelings.
>
> (Hall 1997, 1)

Elaine Scarry (1985) argued that pain occludes language, and she is quite right, but only if one works from the position that language is limited to the spoken and written word. However, if one situates oneself semiotically, then signs and sign-symbols bring pain into existence. These signs define and express pain, categorizing pain so that different broad categories of pain are demarcated, such as emotional, mental, physical, or existential pain (although certainly boundaries are porous). Along with different categories of pain are differing sensations of pain such as burning, aching, sharp, pounding, dull; likewise, there can be movement of pain, radiating or localized, and time of pain, intermittent or chronic. Pain coming into existence through language does not make pain an illusion or an untruth; pain comes into existence through and within social systems, just as the body does and humans do.

Unlike Elaine Scarry (1985) and others (e.g., Coakley, 2007) who take pain to be a phenomenon, one that is outside of language, and indeed escapes our semiotic systems altogether, I contend that pain is a sign subject to conventionality, an analysis/argument I will turn to shortly. But before I do, I want to discuss briefly Peirce's semiotics and his indexical sign, drawing on Umberto Eco, Thomas Sebeok, and Robert Yelle's.

Charles Sanders Peirce

Charles Sanders Peirce (1839–1914) defined a sign as:

> Something which stands to somebody for something in some respect or capacity. It addresses somebody, that is, creates in the mind of that person an equivalent sign, or perhaps a more developed sign. That sign which it creates I call the interpretant of the first sign. The sign stands for something, its object. It stands for that object, not in all respects, but in reference to a sort of idea, which I have called the ground of the *representamen*.
>
> (Peirce in Chandler 2007, 29)

We read in this passage a number of important concepts concerning the sign that were significant to the development Peirce's theory of the sign: the object, the representamen and the interpretant. For example, in the sign "hat" there is an object which is a head covering of different kinds, the representamen which is the sign initiated in response to the object (or first sign), that is, as Daniel Chandler writes, "the *sense* made of the sign" (Chandler 2007, 29, emphasis original) and the interpretant which is the sign, hat, as it is operative in an epistemological-linguistic community.

In terms of modes of signs, or sign-functions as Umberto Eco prefers,[9] Peirce wrote:

> A sign is an icon, an index, or a symbol. An icon is a sign which would possess the character which renders it significant, even though its object had no existence; such as a lead-pencil streak as representing a geometrical line. An index is a sign which would, at once, lose the character which makes it a sign if its object were removed, but would not lose that character if there were no interpretant. Such, for instance, is a piece of mould with a bullet-hole in it as a sign of a shot; for without the shot there would have been no hole; but there is a hole there, whether anybody has the sense to attribute it to a shot or not. A symbol is a sign which would lose the character which renders it a sign if there were no interpretant. Such is any utterance of speech which signifies what it does only by virtue of its being understood to have that signification.
>
> (Peirce 1991, 239)

The modes of signs, icon, index and symbol although having different sign functions remain signs and therefore exist insofar as they are signs, even if the indexical sign was, as Peirce initially thought, "a fragment torn away from the object" (Peirce 1931–58, 2.231 in Chandler 2007, 42), while "the object 'is necessarily existent'" (Peirce 1931–58, 2.230 in Chandler 2007, 42). As Peirce developed his semiotic theory, he quickly became aware that objects, those things he classified as "existent," were indeed signs themselves leading to what Eco has called "unlimited semiosis." "Therefore," writes Eco, quoting Peirce:

> a sign is "anything which determines something else (its *interpretant*) to refer to an object which itself refers (its *object*) in the same way, the interpretant becoming in turn a sign, and so on *ad infinitum*" (2.300) Thus the very definition of 'sign' implies a process of unlimited semiosis.
>
> (Eco 1979, 69; emphasis original)

Eco enjoins that Peirce's semiotic theory engages events/objects that are neither intentionally emitted nor artificially produced, something not found in Saussurean semiotics wherein "the sign is implicitly regarded as a communicative device taking place between two humans intentionally aiming to communicate or to express something" (Eco 1979, 15). And rather than expunging the "natural" sign as he argues Saussurean semioticians do, Eco includes the "natural" sign as a sign and, as such, requiring an interpretant (that is a corresponding sign to the first "sign") to be a sign, while natural signs are as much subject to conventionality as so-called artificial signs (ibid., 16–17).

Pain, what might be called a natural sign by some, is an indexical sign in Peirce's theorizing, but this notion of naturalness produced through the indexical sign-function does not preclude pain represented in the symbol function. Thomas Sebeok wrote:

> Once Peirce realized that the utility of his trichotomy was greatly enhanced when, in order to allow for recognition of differences of degrees, not signs but aspects of signs are being classified, he emended his statement thus: 'it would be difficult if not impossible, to instance an absolute pure index, or to find any sign devoid of the indexical quality' (2:306) ...
>
> (Sebeok 1994, 68)

Therefore, sign functions, multiple in their aspects, can exhibit any one or a combination of aspects or modes in signification.

The Indexical Sign

According to Peirce:

> An *index* is a sign which would, at once, lose the character which makes it a sign if its object were removed, but would not lose that character if there were no interpretant. Such, for instance, is a piece of mould with a bullet-hole in it as sign of a shot; for without the shot there would have been no hole: but there is a hole there, whether anybody has the sense to attribute it to a shot or not.
>
> (Peirce 1991, 239-240)

The indexical sign-function does not impute a direct connection to the object even if described as contiguous with its object, that is, "'whose relation to their objects consists in a correspondence of fact'" (Peirce in Sebeok 1994, 65). The relationship is rhetorical and draws on the metonymical function to provide this sense of contiguity. Indexical signs also have "'the being of present experience'" (ibid., 63), and "furnish positive assurance of the nearness and reality of their Objects. But with the assurance there goes no insight into the nature of those Objects" (Peirce 1991, 251-252).

In terms of its object, the indexical sign does not share characteristics with it, nor is it similar. Rather, Peirce explains:

> it is in dynamical (including spatial) connection with the individual object, on one hand, and with the senses or memory of the person whom it serves as a sign, on the other hand. Let it be recalled that all objects, on the one hand, and the memory being the reservoir of interpretants, on the other hand, are also kinds of signs or systems of signs.
>
> (Peirce in Sebeok 1994, 65)

Peirce also spoke to the qualities of signs, insofar as there a firstness, secondness and thirdness related to the modes of signs. The indexical sign is located in the "mode of being called secondness" "the mode of being of that which is such as it is, with respect to a second but regardless of any third" (Peirce 1986, 639). Firstness is "feeling," immediacy, existence "without recognition or analysis," secondness is that which is there, that intrudes and pushes in, "an external fact, of another something," while thirdness the "synthetic consciousness binding time together, sense of learning, thought" (Peirce 1991, 185). The quality of secondness is one of experience, but experience understood to be equally a part of our linguistic systems. Peirce explains that "[e]xperience generally is what the course of life has compelled me to think" (1986, 640). That is, experience too is a sign and therefore constructed, as Joan Scott (1992) has argued.

In this formulation, the English words such as cue, clue, symptom, and so forth are indexical signs insofar as they point to, provide information on, or register an event or its passing. Indexical signs are verbal signs such as "this" or "that," but they are also olfactory, visual, and gestural and indeed include all aspects of "being" or embodiment. Peirce's classic example of the indexical sign and secondness is the footprint Robinson Crusoe finds in the sand on his deserted island registering the presence of another being and informing him that the being is like him, a human, and as such the sign as index shifts to sign as symbol when Crusoe calls that being a "human" (Peirce 1991, 252).

Applied to pain, pain as indexical sign-function is taken to be a "symptom" while symptom is defined as a "subspecies" of the indexical sign; that is symptoms are "unwitting indexes interpretable by their receivers without the actuality of any intentional sender" (Sebeok 1994, 49). Pain is something that appears to invade our bodies and we are forced to give it our complete attention and, like the wind that moves the weathercock, our bodies are equally moved by pain.

The index and icon sign functions, Robert Yelle writes, "are partly "motivated" signs insofar as the association between them and what they signify is not purely conventional, unlike the vast majority of words [that is symbols]" (2013, 29–30). However, as Yelle rightly notes, "all signs are complex and fall into more than one of these categories" (ibid., 29), and although this may appear to be a contradiction it is not. Since the icon, index and symbol are modes or aspects of signs, or sign functions as Eco calls them, the indexical sign can be motivated, but when a symbol it is not. An example, the footprint of Friday is an indexical sign registering the presence of another being on the island, a trace of their passing, but when Crusoe further interprets the sign to be that of a "human" (man in the text) the symbolic aspect of the sign is present, while the indexical aspect has receded to the background. If we regard signs as aspects, modes or sign functions, the inherent shifting integral for a sign to be a sign, is made visible. Signs are neither fixed nor static, but constantly in a state of flux, shifting as the context shifts. When Yelle uses the concept of the indexical icon with regard to magic, ritualized and/or formulaic, he makes apparent how two aspects of the sign are in primary play in the poetic discourse of magic (ibid.).

In what follows I want to argue that the sign "pain" is an indexical sign, but also it is a symbol, so an indexical symbol, or a sign shifting between both modes and aspects. In the Peircean frame a symbol is "a sign which would lose the character which renders it a sign if there were no interpretant" (1991, 240). The symbol as sign is subject to interpretation; that is, it relies on the functions of representamen and interpretant and therefore is completely subject to convention. Sebeok wrote that "[a] sign without either similarity [icon] or contiguity [index], but only with a conventional link between its signifier and its denotata, and with an intentional class for its designatum, is called a symbol" (1994, 33).

Symbols are also understood to be arbitrary, a quality not associated with the indexical and iconic aspects of the sign in the Peircean frame, as the latter two are seen to be partially motivated insofar as there is a proposed link between the "object" and its signification. For example, the indexical sign of the wind as it moves the weathercock is said to be motivated in that the wind blowing or not blowing is indexed by the movement or lack of movement respectively. Another example is that of folding in rocks due to tectonic stresses. The folds one sees in the rocks of the Rocky Mountains are there whether or not there is a corresponding interpretant that identifies and understands such marks as folds and due to tectonic stresses: the indexical sign function is in play registering the curved line as fold in the rock; the iconic sign-function is in play when all such curved lines in rock are the folding of rocks under extreme pressures, while the symbolic aspect comes into play when the interpretant gathers up the index and icon to signify chevron or a type of rock folding that is a narrow and pointed. The compression marks on the rocks as indexical sign is seen to be motivated insofar as the indexical aspect of the sign is in direct relation with its "object" (but again even our object is a sign). Umberto Eco, however, argues that arbitrariness and motivation are incidental to semiotic theory since a theory of codes is "only concerned with the fact that a convention exists which correlates a given expression [signifier] to a given content [signified], irrespective of the way in which the correlation is posited and accepted" (Eco 1979, 121). As mentioned, for Eco signs are not types, they are sign functions:

a sign function is realized when two functives (expression and content) enter into mutual correlation; the same functive can also enter into another correlation, thus becoming a different functive and therefore giving rise to a new sign-function. Thus signs are the provisional result of coding rules which establish transitory correlations of elements, each of these elements being entitled to enter—under given coded circumstances—into another correlation and thus form a new sign.

(Eco 1979, 49)

It is the flexibility of Eco's combination and development of Saussure and Peirce that allows for a semiotics of pain.

Pain, the Body, and the Indexical and Symbolic Sign Functions

The body too is subject to semiotics and is a sign in the signifying system. Although some would call the body a natural symbol, the category of natural is highly problematic insofar as it assumes a nature/culture dichotomy when we know this dichotomy is a sign function itself in linguistic systems wherein boundaries are generated for a multitude of purposes. The sign functions of the body are complex and elaborate playing out in philosophy, biology, medicine, and feminist theory and so forth, as well as central to many kinds of ritual (rites of passage in particular), central to cosmogonic and anthropogonic myths and frequently represented through symbol. The indexical aspect of the body as sign is the individual body, whatever and whoever that body may be. As indexically signified it is a particular body, but as iconic it is the flesh (also a sign) formulated as body, however that body is signified, that is the plant, animal, insect, etc. body, and as symbol it speaks in many different ways with both negative and positive values attributed to it. For example, we can have the sign of the human body in juxtaposition with other primate bodies to signified difference as simply difference with no imposed value or as more evolved (so plus for humans and negative for other primates). In this play the human body as sign is simultaneously iconic (human body), indexical (*Homo sapiens* as species compared with other primate species) and symbolic (multitude of significations such as more evolved).

Linked to the view that the body is constructed and a sign is the idea that it is also performed; that is the iconic-indexical-symbolic sign-functions of the body and indexical-symbolic sign functions of pain require that they be performed to signify within semiotic systems. To say something is performed is not to say it is or is not authentic. The idea of authentic or inauthentic has no place in semiotics; rather, a semiotic analysis of the body and pain as sign-functions means they are "no longer reified as 'referents,' and ... stand a chance of being opened up ..." (Butler 1993, 29).[10]

That the body and pain are signs and performed does not mean that they are not experiential. Certainly we experience the body and pain in, through and related to flesh, sinew and bone. However, what I argue is that the experience of pain is formed and mapped through knowledge systems of pain (cultural units in Eco's theory: Eco 1979, 166; ideas in Peirce's theory), and therefore subject to conventionality, or a discursive formation of pain. In my own experience of pain, pain invaded and took up lodging in my body, and my effort, then, was to manipulate (e.g., medical treatment, medicine, meditation, breathing exercises, knowledge) my body in order to vanquish or at the very least mitigate *the* pain. The understanding of pain—as that which comes to inhabit the body—locates pain outside and as an object that overtakes and potentially subsumes one erroneously makes it an object.

It is not necessarily that one believes pain is an actual thing in the world, although certainly many treat it as a phenomenon and therefore having concrete status. But this concreteness or realness is an aspect of the indexical sign function. The sense of concreteness implied by the indexical sign function has shaped the discursive formation of pain in such a way as to "produces as an *effect* of its own procedure ... that it nevertheless and simultaneously claims to discover as that which *precedes* its own actions" (Butler 1993, 30). Yelle very nicely illustrates this idea of "realness" with regard to ritual when he writes, "[t]here is a substitution or sleight-of-hand that allows cultural signs—such as language—to be taken as natural, or even consubstantial with physical reality" (2013, 30). It is this interpretation of pain as "real" or as having a causal relation between an actual "object" and the sign that I seek to trouble in this text.

There are numerous ways that pain plays out in the symbol function: narratively, visually, and auditorily, such as seen in Mel Gibson's 2004 *The Passion of the Christ*. Gibson's film reveled in significations of pain: multiple and continuous moments of pain combined to establish pain as the primary signifier in the story of the film's protagonist Jesus. Pain also figures as a primary signifier in ritual, particularly rites of passage where indexically pain is signified and symbolically pain then speaks to overcoming, enduring, or succumbing, to name but a few of its significations. It can signify as the certain path to truth, as when played out in relation to torture (e.g., DuBois 1991; Silverman 2001), as that which purifies (e.g., Glucklich 2001), as that which seasons (e.g., Herdt 1994), as that which bares and exposes (e.g., Burstyn 1999), as a call to serve saints (e.g., Danforth 1989), the significations are legion.

As Elaine Scarry (1985) argued, pain escapes language, and what she says is viable, but only if one works from the position that pain is a phenomenon that precedes the sign. However, if one orients analyses semiotically, it becomes apparent that the indexical and symbolic sign functions bring pain into existence and participate in the production of discourses of pain. Signs define and express pain, and categorize pain providing variant categories and classes of pain such as emotional, mental, physical, or existential (although certainly boundaries between these kinds of pain are porous) or measurements such as scales wherein levels of pain are quantified. Along with different kinds of pain are differing sensations of pain such as burning, aching, sharp, pounding, dull, there can be movement of pain, radiating or localized, and time of pain, intermittent or chronic. Pain coming into existence through our semiotic systems does not make pain an illusion or an untruth; rather, pain has no meaning outside of our semiotic systems.

Discursive Constructions of Pain: Myth, Ritual, and Sign-symbol

My interest in pain and the discourses that shape it is primarily directed toward interpreting pain in the representational narratives of myth, ritual and symbol (the latter I refer to as sign-symbol). In each of these narratives, pain is made to signify in a multitude of ways and equally intersects with other signs, such as gender/sex, race and indigeneity, class, sexuality, humanity, power, truth, and deceit, etc. to name a few. Pain, when intersecting with other signs can take a secondary role, such as when it is used to define a proper masculinity, or it can take a primary role, such as when in torture it intersects with "truth" in order to produce "the truth."

For example, René Descartes declared, if contentiously, that animals lacked reason and indeed consciousness and therefore lacked the capacity for deep sensory perception, including that of pain (Descartes 1924).[11] Clearly Descartes was in error, but he was of course invested in establishing a boundary between the human (actually "man") and the non-human animal in the grand design of existence initiated and overseen by the Christian deity. Indeed, the practice of vivisection on living conscious animals was a method used by Descartes and adopted by others in the period. For Descartes, pain was a rational experience and if animals did not reason, as demonstrated by their lack of speech, then certainly they did not feel pain (see also Kalof 2007). In Descartes's view pain is an experience of "mankind" only, and therefore a signification of being human in relation to deity, while the lack of pain marked the "animal," and all those likened to the animal; those other so-called brutes[12] marked by race and geopolitical location in the onslaught of colonization. Indeed, the term "brute" gained in popularity having been applied to those marked by race or class. These so-called unrefined humans felt little pain, and indeed the extensive and unremitting use of pain was a necessity in order to control those redefined as "brutes," "natives," "mules," "savages," "squaws," "slaves," and so forth as Eurowestern countries and then later as nations swarmed the globe.

Certainly Descartes was by no means an intentional mythographer, but his philosophy was replete with mythemes,[13] such as reason acting as the yellow brick road to deity, that non-human animals lacking reason (following Aristotle) were incapable of feeling pain, since they could not understand pain, or that non-human animals were automata (see Anita Guerrini 1989). The subjection of non-human animals (and human animals in some cases) to vivisection, scientific experiments such as injections of vitriol, transfusion (animal to animal and animal to human), and a plethora of other horrors (ibid., 395ff) were made sensible by Descartes's mechanistic philosophy which contextually acted to allow such a view to make sense. In Descartes's discursive framing of pain, pain acted as a truth to signify what is human and what is not.

Ritual, like myth, also contributes to a discursive formation of pain. In ritual, pain acts as a means by which to cross a threshold in rites of passage, or pain is the medium by which whatever powers that be, e.g., saints, orisha, deities, energies, ancestors and so forth, communicate with humans. Pain also communicates power, and those who inflict pain speak their power to those on whom pain is inflicted. Much the same as vivisection was justified by reference to "man's" power over non-human animals, so too torture is a ritual act whereby the powerful demonstrate their power through painful inscription upon the flesh of those marked as lesser, as other, as non-human.

In rites of passage such as male and female circumcision wherein the flesh is cut away in order to mark a transition into adulthood, pain is a central component. The cut as indexical sign function is important since it identifies the transition, while pain as sign-symbol signifies as the threshold of this transition marking a movement from one way of being to another (see Gilbert Herdt's work with the Sambia people, 1994).

In ritual, the application and expression of pain to the body are a visual event that speaks the "truth" of pain, even as it speaks the "truth" of the system of belief and practice. Ritual, an embodied discourse, uses the body to provide a canvas of pain whereby pain is given concrete existence in the body. In Tiv scarification, for example, pain is traced upon the body in the extensive tattooing performed on young women coming of age.[14] Bruce Lincoln's text, *Emerging from the Chrysalis* (1981), provides some discussion on this event. In scarification the young woman's belly is incised by the artist using a razor with a line running from the throat to the navel. Around the navel concentric circles are incised into her flesh. The basic design of line and circles is further enhanced with other kinds of patterns. Once the cuts (indexical sign-function) are made, charcoal is rubbed into them (ibid., 34–39). Whether pain is central to Tiv scarification, certainly pain is an aspect of the ritual play and that pain has left traces on the body. These traces, patterned in numerous ways, are understood to enhance the beauty of the young woman (ibid., 35) so that in Tiv scarification we have beauty and pain linked together, a frequent motif in many cultures. The traces of pain etched on her body, a sign-symbol, not only speak to aspects of the system of belief and practice, such as time, genealogy, relations to the land and so forth (ibid., 48–49), but also to pain which is given concrete and permanent representation on the bodies of young Tiv women who practiced the ritual.

The representation of pain in visual media very much presents a language of pain. For example, images of the crucifixion in some forms of Christianity, especially the Catholic Christianity of Mexico and Latin and South America, emphasize the torture and pain of their deity on the cross, and indeed even the whipping, carrying and hanging from the cross of their deity are enacted in ritual pageants by Christian brotherhoods. Here the torment of deity graphically represented on a crucifix or enacted through ritual shapes and codes pain: it visually speaks the pain and those who look upon this visual representation understand the language. This is certainly a discourse that Mel Gibson developed in his graphic 2004 film *The Passion of the Christ*.

The visual discourse of pain is something seen from the earliest representations of human groups (e.g., Lascaux) until the present in numerous media formats. The representation of pain would appear to be a favorite and frequent motif. Although Georges Bataille's text, *The Tears of Eros* (1989), is concerned with eroticism; he, like all good theorists of the Marquis de Sade, brings pain and pleasure into close relationship. In this text Bataille examines representations of eroticism from the ancient Greeks to the modern world of Europe, and emergent in many is the mixing of pain and pleasure. In the images Bataille chose we clearly see a fascination with an effort to capture pain, pain as torment and often torture as evidenced in Lucas Cranach's *The Saw* (ibid., 88) or in the photographs of the torture called the "Hundred Pieces" (ibid., 204–206). Bataille found the photograph fascinating and he would look at it daily. Reflecting on such a horrific image of pain prompted him to ask: "I wonder what the Marquis de Sade would have thought of this image, Sade who dreamed of torture, which was inaccessible to him, but who never witnessed an actual torture session?" (ibid., 206).

In the above discussion my effort has been to destabilize the category of pain arguing that it is not a natural category, although certainly it is an embodied category. But because pain emerges from the body does not mean that it cannot be discursive, for the body is also produced in discourse. But neither is pain simply an external discourse interpellated (to draw on Louis Althusser); it is also an internal discourse shaped in and through our bodies. Following the arguments of George Lakoff and Mark Johnson in their text *Philosophy in the Flesh* (Lakoff and Johnson 1999), then, I must account for the embodied knowledge mapped as it is through our neurological systems. Although I do not mean to track pain through neurological systems per se, since I am not invested in finding the truth of pain, thinking of embodiment as being in the flesh means understanding that the flesh shapes discourse even as it is shaped by discourse. They argue: "The mind is inherently embodied. Thought is mostly unconscious. Abstract concepts are largely metaphorical" (ibid., 3). I certainly do not disagree with Lakoff and Johnson's statements, although I reject philosophical realism, even the "embodied kind" that shapes their work (ibid., 25). However, their third statement I find most valuable for the kind of work I wish to develop with regard to the discursive formation of pain, one that will of necessity be cognizant of a history of pain, and its human, gender/sex, race, class, and geopolitical encoding.

Both pain and the body have been central to systems of belief and practice and therefore to myth, ritual and sign-symbol. These representational narratives provide a concreteness to pain; a concreteness that represents pain as a thing in the world. This kind of conceptualization takes pain beyond the boundaries of a human body so that we may speak of pain as something that overcomes us, brings us down, takes us by surprise and so forth. Pain exists "out there" even as it is only found "in here," and it is this kind of conceptualization of pain that needs to be disrupted.

Both sign functions (pain and the body) have been and continue to be central to systems of belief and practice and therefore to myth, ritual and sign-symbol. The representational narratives of myth, ritual and sign-symbol engage pain and the body robustly and in so doing add to the indexical aspect or mode, the outcome of which obscures pain and the body as sign functions and instead proposes both to be phenomena. These narratives conceptualize pain as beyond the boundaries of human "culture" and inhabiting the wilds of "nature" or the realm of demons, deities, and animals. Pain as an indexical-symbolic sign function has eluded many as those in medicine try to quantify and/or image it; those in the military control or apply it; while the rest of us simply try to avoid "it." Pain, like all sign functions, "produces as an *effect* of its own procedure ... that it nevertheless and simultaneously claims to discover as that which *precedes* its own actions" (Butler 1993, 30, emphasis original).

Chapter 2

Mythic Caesura, Pain, and the Boundary between Non-human and Human Animals

> The question of our proper relationship to other animals is a question with a long history—as long as the history of our species. Throughout history and in all places, animals have been an important part of human culture. They have been hunted, domesticated, befriended and eaten, worshiped and feared, romanticized and demonized, studied and mythologized. Reflections upon our relationships with them have been continuous and are expressed in our traditions, arts, literature, religion and sciences.
>
> (Mack 1999, xvi)

Introduction

One of the primary ways by which I engage my work in the study of systems of belief and practice is the analysis of discourse. Discourses can be numerous things, but generally they are conceptualizations deployed through our signing systems. Our signing systems, language, art, engraving and architecture, sign-symbols, media, gesture, and so forth are the ways by which our "existence" is effected (brought into existence), encoded and given meaning. Michel Foucault (1972, 1980a) and subsequently Stuart Hall (1997), Judith Butler (1993), and Chris Weedon (2001), among others, laid out the process of analyzing discourse included which is the discomposing of those things we take to be normative and natural demonstrating how a concept, animals for example, is constructed, shaped, and maintained through discourse. For example, the notion of homosexuality, and therefore heterosexuality, was shown by Foucault to have emerged in the eighteenth century of Europe, or again when Thomas Laqueur (1992) demonstrated how the notion of male and female as a naturally derived opposition of sexes emerged at the turn of the nineteenth century of the Eurowest. Previously the taken for granted knowledge, under the influence of Aristotle among others, represented the female and male as sharing the same sex but different genders; however, the female was misbegotten—a lesser and inverted version of the male.

To do the work of decomposing, Michel Foucault (1978), for example, looked at various discourses in Western Europe from the sixteenth to early twentieth centuries produced in French Catholicism, medicine, philosophy, emergent biology, legal texts, and governmental policy in order to show how sexuality, as such, became a subject in and through discourse and how that discourse shaped it. In his work he demonstrated how sexuality began to be signified as both a threat and a possibility, but as such required strict control in order that threat be averted and possibility achieved. He showed how heterosexual vaginal intercourse within the bond of marriage was determined to be the only proper, that is morally and legally, form of sex (Foucault 1978, 37–39). Sex outside of marriage was deemed both criminal and sinful (full of sin), while masturbation was seen to be sinful and unhealthy, leading both the "soul" and the body into illness (ibid., 44). In this instance Eurowestern medicine and a broad-based Christianity came together to shape a discursive formation of sex and sexuality as dangerous and in need of external control and guidance (ibid., 104). Assumed in this understanding was a belief that human beings left to their own devices—particularly those segments of the social body marked as unreasoning—could potentially revert to their "animal" or "baser" nature (behave like "beasts" or non-human animals lacking the ideal human quality of rationality).

A literary example of this fear of devolution to the "beast" that is contained and controlled by the use of reason can be seen in the novel *The Strange Case of Dr. Jekyll and Mr. Hyde* (Stevenson 2004). Written in 1886 by Robert Louis Stevenson, the novella relates the tale of a doctor who through (unauthorized) experimentation reverts to a "beast": Mr. Hyde is immensely violent; stealing, raping, and murdering at will. Mr. Hyde is a being operating fully in a "nature red in tooth and claw" to quote Alfred Tennyson's poem "In Memoriam A.H.H." (1849), and although Stevenson's story (and Tennyson's poem) precedes Darwin's *The Origin of the Species* published in 1859 (Darwin 1963) and *The Descent of Man* published in 1871 (Darwin 1981), certainly Darwinists took up the phrase to express Darwin's evolutionary theory of natural selection. One of the notions that emerged in relation to Charles Darwin's theories, propounded not by Darwin, but by social Darwinists, was the idea of devolution or evolution in reverse. Stevenson's novel speaks to this fear, as does Rudyard Kipling's short story "The mark of the beast" written in 1890. Such views of non-human and human animals distort Darwin's insight that humans are animals as well.[1]

Non-human and Human Animals

Living beings construct knowledge whereby they establish a world, an *Umwelt* that is knowable to them. These knowledge systems precede any one being and consequently beings are brought into knowledge systems and constructed by, in and through it, even as they contribute, challenge, and/or deconstruct their received knowledge. Knowledge is never fixed and is constantly shifting in tune with the context from which it emerges making apparent the instability of what we think we know. If knowledge can be destabilized, then so too the fixity and certainty of the sign of the "human." One way to destabilize the sign of the human is to mark its relationship with the animal and by doing so I can see that the signs "human" and "animal" work in conjunction with each other to define something since they are invested with signification beyond the words human and animal, and speak of something larger; among other things, a significant binary relationship between the two that establishes ontological and metaphysical boundaries and moral and ethical values.

To destabilize a natural boundary and mark the relationship between animals and humans, I use the terms non-human animals and human animal. The idea of a natural boundary is central to both signs, and like the so-called opposition between the signs of female/feminine and male/masculine there is nothing natural about it. Rather, like the binary of female/feminine and male/masculine providing logic to the mytheme Man the hunter, woman the gatherer, the binary of animal and human provides logic to the mytheme of "the servants of humanity" along with the deities, as I discuss further on when engaging the texts *Iliad* and *Popul Vuh*. From the outset in this chapter, then, I work to destabilize the binary and reframe the relationship so that animal is linked to human even as it is a "non"-human animal, while human is linked to animal, that is human animal. My effort is to make apparent that the signs of animal and human are constructed within and through human linguistic systems and further, are constructed by and with binary logic both of which secure the value of human animals over non-human animals in existence. This binary system is invaluable to racist, xenophobic, colonialist, and other oppressive systems in our social bodies.

Having situated the location of the animal/human in the social (and not in nature) what is equally evident is that value, as in all binaries, is ascribed to the binary pair so that the animal carries negative value (–) and the human positive value (+) in their ontological, epistemological and metaphysical relationships.[2] Although the phrase non-human and human animals continues to privilege the human and mark a difference between the two, my first effort is simply to recognize that the human animal produces discourses reflecting on themselves and others, while the second, the use of "non" is an effort to call forth the knowledge that humans are animals as much as animals are animals.

If I understand the signs of animal and human operate in a binary system, then I am positioned to ask what other binaries might be linked with this one to form a binary set, which through metaphorical (as one is to the other) and metonymical (as one stands in relation to the other) functions allow the operation of the binary (see also Juschka 2009). In the binary set below, for example, we can see how otherfication established in the animal/human binary can act as a basis for marking as "other" those deemed "not the same" within a social body. The metaphorical relationship establishes links among concepts in a set,[3] for example, animal is to nature, is to savage, is to irrational and so on down the list, even as the metonymical relationship ensures a normative linking of the two concepts, that is animal evokes human, as nature evokes culture, and down the list.[4]

(-)	(+)
animal	human
nature	culture
savage	civilized
irrational	rational
superstition	religion
native	European
black	white
female	male
feminine	masculine
negative	positive

The Animal–Human Binary in Eurowestern Knowledge Systems

Having made visible the binary opposition of animal–human, I now want to briefly discuss the historical development of this binary in three discursive formations; scientific, Christian, and philosophical-political, the last really a discussion of the development of the sign of "man"; and I use man advisedly here as this sign is masculine, white, and Eurowestern and is a construct that supports and upholds the truth of both Enlightenment scientific and Christian narratives.

Science is the epistemological foundation of the Eurowest and was an effect/outcome of the European Enlightenment, which coincided with the rise of capitalism and modernity (early to mid-seventeenth century) and intersects with emergent Protestant Christianities (mid-sixteenth century) during the period of the Protestant Reformation. The Romantic period or Romanticism (eighteenth century) followed the Enlightenment and sought to challenge its rationalism and within this, its mechanistic view. In the elevated view of "man" (in this instance white, Eurowestern, and masculine) and his link to deity and overcoming of "nature"; something we see in art, literature, music, and so forth, non-human animals are lowered and ultimately condemned. Proposed by René Descartes (1596–1650) in early modernity, and based on Aristotle's *Generation of Animals*, was the idea that animals were different than humans because the latter (specifically proper adult male citizens of the polis in the instance of Aristotle) had a rational soul and could reason, while the former could not; they lacked (–) what the human supposedly had: a rational soul and a capacity to reason (Aristotle 1979). The answer, then, to what is the "human" or what is "mankind"? was(is) determined by defining it as "that which is" (+) over and against that which is not (–). For example, a cup is defined as an object that holds, typically, fluids allowing one to drink from it, while the human or "man" has no definition other than what it *is* in relation to that which it *is not*. According to the *Merriam-Webster Dictionary*, human is "characteristic of or relating to man in his essential nature … relating to, or resembling man or his attributes in distinction from the lower animals … to be human is to understand, to evaluate, to choose, to accept responsibility" (2000) – in other words, to reason. And if in science "men" were no longer animals, this was because they had transcended the instincts and via evolution had risen above their animalistic state through the development of reason, tool making, altruism, language, signing systems, cognition, and so on.

These views are some of the means by which "speciesism," or the positive valuation of one species, in this instance *Homo sapiens*, over other species, and indeed, all forms of life and non-life on the planet, is enacted. Cary Wolfe, in his text *Animal Rites: American Culture, the Discourse of Species and Posthumanist Theory* (2003a) comments that Sigmund Freud's (1856–1939) theory of the origin of *Homo sapiens*, having read as well Charles Darwin, locates the shift from animal to human in the "act of 'organic repression' whereby they begin to walk upright and rise above life on the ground among blood and feces":

> These formerly exercised a sexually exciting effect but now, with "the diminution of the olfactory stimuli," they seem disgusting, leading in turn to what Freud calls a "cultural trend toward cleanliness" and creating the "sexual repression" that results in the "founding of the family and so to the threshold of human civilization."
>
> (Wolfe 2003a, 2)

As Wolfe comments, by privileging vision over and above any of the other senses, in this instance smell or the olfactory sense, Sigmund Freud, among others, assumes a normative hierarchical organization of senses using non-human animals by which to develop it. Non-human animals (−) were (and continue to be) considered to be inferior to humans (+) and have less life value. As such, then, senses they favor must signify as animalistic, while humans, on the other hand, have over the centuries favored sight, which must then signify as human: both sight and the human are privileged reinforcing view of a natural hierarchy that defined life, and the special place human animals occupied. It is clear that the binary of animal–human shaped Freud's thought, and indeed his assumption reflects Eurowestern science's certainty that the human animal has a special place in existence, while this view is also reflected in the majority of systems of belief and practice central to the organization of social bodies in the Eurowest (on this subject of the distinction between human and animal, see also, among others, Agamben 2004, 1998; Haraway 2003; Ingold 2000, 1988; Midgley 1995).

The Animal–Human Binary in Systems of Belief and Practice

This leads me to the animal–human binary in a broad-based Christianity. Now I say broad-based since there are multiple Christianities operating in the Eurowest, along with other systems of belief and practice such as Islams, Judaisms, various and sundry spiritualities, folks systems and so forth (including variation in historical manifestations as well), and it is the combination of their monotheisms that tend to dominate metaphysical, epistemological and ontological views. Grounded in this broad-based Christianity is an ontology wherein the human animal is separated from other animals by and through having a special and unique relationship with deity (or group of three deities). This notion of uniqueness is drawn from Genesis 1:26-27, which is the primary anthropogonic myth in Christianity, wherein deity creates humankind "in our image" and then proceeds in 1:28 to give humans dominion over all life. The narrative assumes a hierarchical structure, wherein those below are ruled by those above. This structure is emphasized in the works of some significant thinkers who influenced the shape of Christianity such as the Pauline letters, and the writings of Jerome, Augustine, and Aquinas, all of whom were influenced by Platonic and Aristotelian ontologies. Furthermore, this normative hierarchical view is evidenced in what was called "the great chain of being" or the understanding that the value of a thing's being is defined by their location on a vertical continuum, with top (closest to deity) having the greatest value and bottom the least value (furthest from deity).

The notion of the great chain of being was fully developed in medieval period and can be seen in the early modern drawing of Didacus Valades's *Rhetorica Christiana* (Figure 1). We see in the image that deity represents the

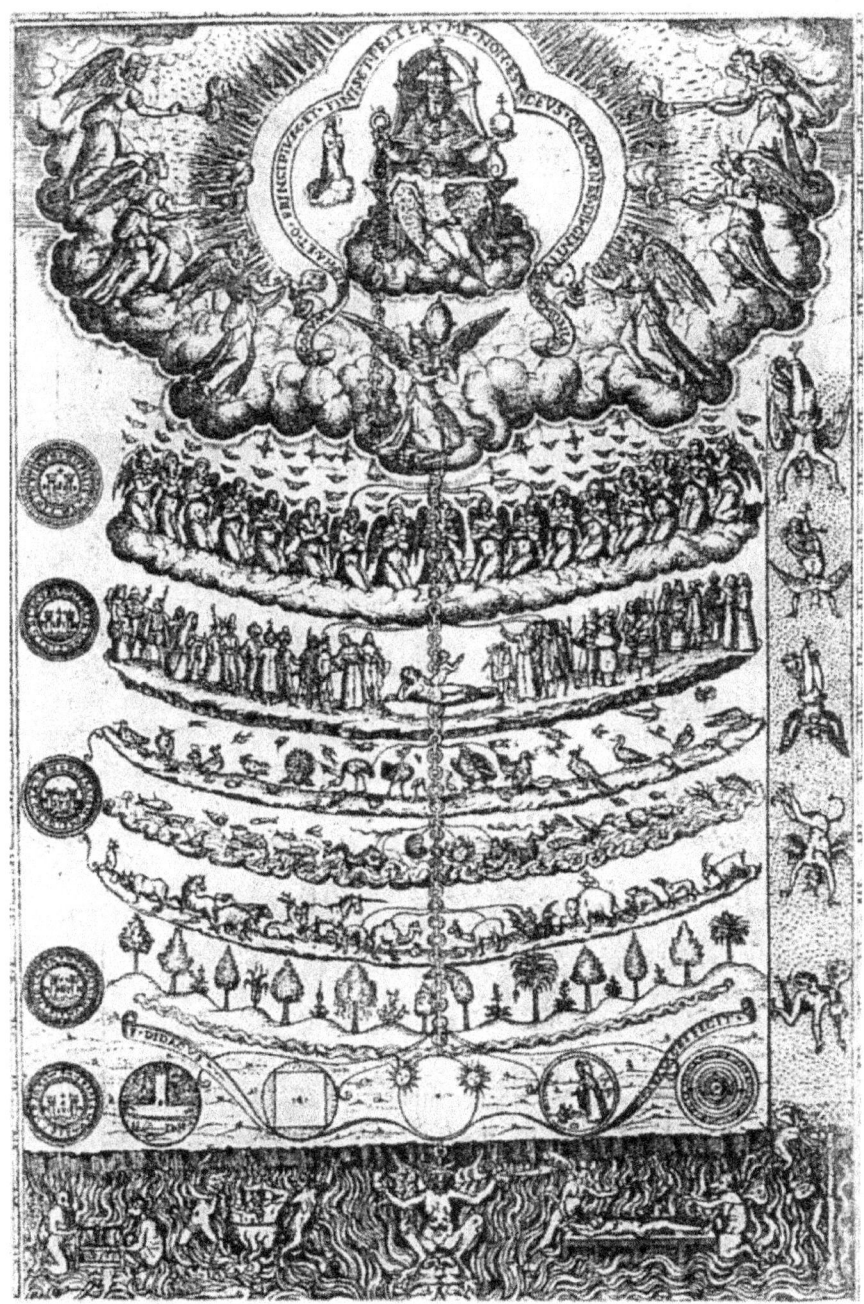

Figure 1. Didacus Valades's *Rhetorica Christiana*.

ideal of being and each level down is a movement away from the ideal to the base, rock, wherein there is no "being." Above rocks are plants which exist and live, next up are animals which have existence, life, motion, and appetite, above these humans are located, then angels and finally deity. There are further divisions within each of these large groups, so that for example, gold is higher than mere rock, the oak tree is higher than the demonic Yew tree, wild animals over domestic animals, with the lion located at the top of wild animals, while dogs and horses are above sheep and cows, male above female, king above peasant, and archangel above cherubim.[5]

A primary aspect of this vertical chain of being that provides its own values is the body-flesh/soul-spirit binary, a central and significant binary in Christianities. In this blueprint of life, developed along moralistic and valuative lines (as all binaries are), the human animal has a soul (+), in Aristotle's (1979) terms a rational soul, something non-human animals lack being only body (-). In Christian terms, this came to mean that animals lacked a soul, and, as is noted in the second anthropogonic myth found in Genesis 2, deity breathes life into "his" ultimate creation, Adam, but does not provide this breath of life to non-human animals (or Eve for that matter).

This kind of understanding of non-human animals shaped how science, philosophy, social-political systems, and people in general understand themselves and non-human animals. This great chain of being is a conceptualization that continues to hold sway in Eurowestern (for example see factory farms, experimental research using live non-human animals, dog shows and fights, horse races, hunting, circuses, road-side zoos, marine parks, humane societies, and so forth) ontology or being in the world.

Certainly, systems of belief and practice were/are central sites for the discursive formation of ontological difference invested in establishing non-human animals as lower or lesser than human animals; and indeed, much thought and ink has been spent establishing a boundary between the two. This value-laden boundary is a product of the animal–human binary, which often, but not always, works in tandem with the nature–culture binary. In this binary play, non-human animals are metaphorically linked to nature, while other binaries can be brought to bear to establish a set, for example, female–male, child–adult, native–colonizer, sorcerer–religious, savage–civilized, feral–domestic, wild–tame and demonic–angelic.

But systems of belief and practice were/are also instrumental toward challenging the "inhumane" treatment of non-human animals arguing that non-human animals are also part of deity's creation and therefore deserving of care and respect even if inferior (-) to humans. This kind of view can be seen in John Locke's (1632–1704) work wherein, in contradistinction to René

Descartes's view that animals do not feel pain, he argued, in his 1693 piece "Some Thoughts Concerning Education," that animals do have feelings, and that unnecessary cruelty toward them is morally wrong as well as bad for "mankind" as it hardens them (Locke 1975, 130). This view of non-human animals was supported by others like Jean-Jacques Rousseau (1712–1778) and Immanuel Kant (1724–1804); however, they did not consider animals to be on a par with humans. Drawing on this line of philosophical thought, Richard Martin, a member of the British Parliament and the Reverend Arthur Broome (Anglican) established, with others, the Society for the Prevention of Cruelty to Animals, which became a royal society in 1840 (i.e. the RSPCA), having been granted a royal charter.

Animality and Humanity: Marking the Difference

In the following sections, I examine and compare the separation of human and non-human animals in the *Iliad* and *Odyssey* of ancient Greece and the Mayan myth the *Popul Vuh*.[6] Found in the Homeric and Maya texts is a necessity to draw a boundary between the non-human and human animal: a boundary based on kinship relations, speech and bodily differences. In both texts the category of non-human animal acts as the means by which the category of human, less its animal, is constructed. Non-human and human animals signify as separate and distinct, and the unstable boundary between the two serves as a regulatory mechanism to mark outsiders from insiders, while simultaneously establishing vertical structures within the social body. By examining and comparing the mythic play of non-human and human animals (and the boundary between) and their naturalization and/or metaphysicalization, specifically with their intersection with kinship, linguistic capacity, and ultimately the indexical sign of pain, I argue that the sign of pain is used to augment the border between non-human and human animals. I also discuss how the boundary is primary to constructing knowledge about non-human and human animals, and how the sign of the non-human animal is foundational to the veracity of the sign of the human (less its animal). Through the accounting of bodily difference a boundary is drawn, while pain stabilizes the boundary even if the indexical sign can erode the boundary between the non-human and human animals when pain forces them to share an *Umwelt*.

The Ur-other: Non-human Animals

> The division of life into vegetal and relational, organic and animal, animal and human, therefore passes first of all as a mobile border within living man [*sic*],

and without this intimate caesura the very decision of what is human and what is not would probably not be possible.
(Agamben 2004, 15)

Anthropogonic and demogonic myths, myths that speak to the institution of the human and its social body, are central to conceptualizing existence and everything therein. They are foundational myths that in founding something, define it, and in defining it speak to what it is and, more often, what it is not. Because anthropogonic and demogonic kinds of myth are foundational myths, and therefore supportive of the operative episteme,[7] they are often employed in order to shore up, challenge, shift, and/or articulate their respective epistemes (see also Lincoln 1986, 1989; Smith 1982; Waldau and Patton 2006). An often found aspect of anthropogonic myths[8] is a boundary marking a break between human and non-human animals. The primary separation between human and non-human animals, then, acts as a means to set the limits and center for the category of human.

Anthropogonic and demogonic myths, by providing definition, mark boundaries between that which is the same and that which is different. They also speak to the establishing of other kinds of boundaries; gender/sex, status, sexuality and so forth, but for the purposes of this chapter the boundary between the non-human and human animal is focused upon. I do this because the non-human and human animal divide is often significant to other kinds of divides such as those based on gender/sex, race, sexualities, class, and so forth. In order to limit my analysis, I focus on two categorical criteria, the body (related to ontology and in this category kinship and speech) and the body and pain, as they are significant toward establishing a *caesura* as argued by Agamben (2004).

The Iliad and Odyssey: Kinship, Speech, and Normative Boundaries

The authorship and date of the *Iliad* (Homer 1999) and *Odyssey* (Homer 1998) continues to be a contested subject; however, I follow Robert Fowler (2004), among others, and date the earliest versions to around 700 BCE[9] and earlier oral versions to sometime in the 800s BCE. The *Iliad* tells a complex tale of power and those who seemingly have it and those who seemingly do not. Power is never fixed in one location evidenced by the unremitting struggles for power between Hera and Zeus, Apollo and the Greeks, Agamemnon and Achilles, Achilles and Hector, Hector and Andromache, Odysseus and the "low" born Theristes among others. Even as these struggles are played out, a struggle for power between non-human and human animals is not represented indicating that a *fait accompli* concerning the natural and metaphysical subordination of non-human animals (as it was for slaves, women and the so-called low-born). The Homeric texts do not seek to construct or establish a boundary between non-human and human animals; rather difference and boundary are assumed and indeed employed to establish other kinds of boundaries such as between Trojan and Greek, slave and free, feminine and masculine, domestic and wild, low born and highborn, priests and kings, and so on.

Non-human animals are taken to be other from the outset in the Homeric texts even if they share attributes with human animals such as breath, thought, emotion, desire, and ability to communicate (Heath 2005, 48). But even as the sign of the non-human animal appears to overlap with the sign of the human animal, three ontological signifiers marked the difference and thereby secure the boundary between them: kinship, speech and pain. Kinship establishes non-human and human animals as separated by a wide gulf, while speech, following John Heath (2005), is used to mark the so-called uniqueness of the human animal, and linked to humans deities who also share in this capacity. Shared attributes such as breath, thought, and emotion between the human and non-human animal allowed for a connection, but only insofar as it allowed human animals to dominate non-human animals. What such shared attributes did not do was speak to kinship. Rather, shared attributes signified non-human and human animals share in existence.

In the *Iliad* and *Odyssey* the non-human animal occupies a category that is completely separate from the human animal. Shared attributes, mentioned above, speak to an understanding that there is a connection between non-human and human animals, but these shared attributes, breath, thought, emotion, desire, and ability to communicate, allow for rudimentary relations between the two groups, and are not indicative of kinship.[10] This conceptualization of a lack of kinship is evident in several instances where non-human animals play a significant role in the narratives. In book 10 of the *Odyssey*, Odysseus's men ate and drank Circe's poisoned food and subsequently were turned into swine by Circe. But they were not truly swine as "they had the heads, and voice, and bristles, and shape of swine, but their minds [*noos*] remained unchanged, just as they were before" (*Od.* 10.239–241). Bodily swine, the sailors remained inwardly human with a human nature: They had been only masked as swine and were able to resume their human form once the spell was lifted. As Heath wrote, the *noos*, or mind, is the place of reason, and non-human animals are representing as lacking this capacity that is taken to be part of "human nature."

Another myth of transformation, found in Apollodorus (3.4.3), is that of Actaeon turned into a stag by Artemis (in another version Zeus is named as

Actaeon's tormentor). In this tale, as with many others, when humans are turned into animals the outcome is not a happy one: Actaeon, bodily a stag, retains his human mind, but unable to speak, his hunting dogs (Lynceaus, Balios and Amarynthos, and Spartyos, Omargos, and Bores) set upon him and tear him apart. As with Odyssey's men, transition from human animal to non-human animal is superficial, a masking that conceals the human beneath.[11] Non-human and human animals share no kinship and when there is a mixing of the human and non-human animal, the mixing is incomplete and frequently met with violence and death.[12]

In Homer's epics, if non-human animals do not share kinship with human animals, they also do not have the capacity for speech, or rather human speech.[13] Deities, the semi-divine, and the otherworldly all have the capacity for human speech, but non-human animals do not. Circe, "dread goddess of human speech" (δεινὴ θεὸς αὐδήεσσα) (Od. 11.8), removes the capacity for speech from Odysseus's men when she transforms them into swine. Masked as swine and without speech they must live as swine even if their minds and hearts retain their human nature.[14] Further along in book 11 of the Odyssey, Odysseus has agreed to journey to Hades to seek out the advice of the great prophet Tiresias. In this episode Odysseus sacrifices several sheep and a bull to bring the dead to him. As the dead approach, Homer writes they emit "unearthly shrieks" (θεσπεσίῃ ἰαχῇ) (11.43) and will not be able to speak until they have tasted the blood of the sacrifice. Dead, they have lost the capacity of human speech and, instead, like non-human animals they emit unintelligible sounds.[15] Interestingly, it is the blood of the non-human animal that allows for the capacity of speech, which might suggest non-human animal blood has a property that allows those who cannot speak, to speak. It is not, however, a property of non-human animals, rather as sacrifice the non-human animals signify sharing in the realm of deities and in this secure the power of speech for the dead, much as Hera gave Xanthus the capacity to speak.

In the Iliad, a scene that further highlights speech as a criterion to mark a boundary between the human and non-human is that of the interchange between the semi-divine horse Xanthus and hero Achilles. At the end of book 19, as Heath (2005, 39–40) notes, Xanthus is given speech or "human voice" (αὐδήεντα—voiceful) by Hera in order to speak intelligibly to Achilles about the hero's impending death. As soon as the words were out of Xanthus's mouth, however, the Enrinyes or Fates, stopped his voice (αὐδήεν) and Xanthus was silenced. Although an instance of a non-human animal speaking and speaking authoritatively in the text, Xanthus's speech was marked as out of the ordinary, extraordinary, while the reader is informed, Xanthus is no ordinary non-human animal, but one with divine origins having the West wind and the harpy Podarge as parents (*Il.*, 16.150–151). But even divine origins are not enough, and the text ensures that first a deity provides Xanthus with speech and second as quickly as Xanthus was given speech deities removed it: such a thing is, the text comments, against the order of existence. Non-human animals make noises such as barking, grunting, or neighing and although their sounds are certainly taken to be communicative, these sounds are not classified as "speech" as speech by very definition is human. Only deities, humans, the otherworldly and the blood-sated dead partake of speech; non-human animals cannot and should not.

If speech is one criterion to elevate the human, authoritative speech further marks boundaries between human animals, locating some more closely to the non-human animal and others further away. As Heath notes, authoritative speech is only given to men (that is properly masculine men) in the Homeric texts.[16] The narratives are not interested, Heath argues, in differentiating non-human animals and animals *per se*, but more interested in establishing that proper speech, authoritative speech, one that is followed by proper action, belongs to adult men, and not women, children, and slaves. Although these last have speech, their speech carries no authority, they do not have a public voice and therefore cannot "effect" (bring into being) proper action (Heath 2005, 77). Above all are the deities, and their speech in the Homeric texts is the most eloquent and exquisite of all speech. Quoting Heath:

> There is one irrefutable difference between Homeric animals and humans: animals do not speak. Humans, in fact, can barely keep quiet in the epics: about half of each poem comprises characters' speech. This divergence, although not a moral one, forms the basis for a separation of a variety of groups in the Homeric poems, groups that in the classical period will form the core of the "Other" that has been so thoroughly investigated in scholarship over the past few decades. The use and abuse of language becomes a means of differentiation, usually without the moral implications of later times.
>
> (Heath 2005, 51)

Heath also comments that the category of non-human animal, used to nice rhetorical effect in the Homeric texts to speak about human animals, was later drawn upon by the Greeks of classical period and employed as the ground for the sign of the "other": those who are unlike and therefore outside of one's group. In the binary play of other/same, the other is seen as an external, an outside and as outside deficient and often a threat if not properly controlled.

Two scenes played out before the gates of Troy demonstrate othering through the deployment of the boundary between human and non-human animals drawing on the criteria of kinship and speech to do so. At the outset of the scene Greeks and Trojans have met before the walls of Troy:

> Now when they were marshalled, the several companies with their captains, the Trojans came on with clamour and with a cry like birds, even as the clamour of cranes that ariseth before the face of heaven ... But the Achaeans came on in silence, breathing fury, eager at heart to bear aid each man to his fellow.
> (*Iliad* 3.1–9)

In this passage the Trojans are signaled as outsiders, non-Greeks (ironically even as the text situates Greeks as geographical outsiders lingering outside the walls of Troy), when the text analogically links them to non-human animals through the noise—not speech—they emit likened to the "cry of birds" and "clamour of cranes" as they enjoin the battlefield.[17] In another metaphor the multiple languages attributed to the Trojans and their allies by Homer, is likened to the bleating of ewes calling to their lambs, as they waited to be milked having returned from the fields (*Il.* 4.433–438). Juxtaposed with the Trojans are the noiseless Greeks again with their quiet and deadly approach (4.427–432) signally their difference from the animalistic Trojans, and implicitly linking the Greeks to the sign of the human: humans have speech and animals emit meaningless sounds (note also how Ares is linked to the Trojans and Athena to the Greeks associating the Trojans with chaos and confusion and Greeks with order and sense).

The use of non-human animals to signify otherness throughout book 3 of the *Iliad* is Paris, who sports a panther skin on his shoulders, does not appear to have control of speech, and indeed is represented as lacking authoritative speech, not surprising considering his panther skin. In Paris's first speech act of book 3, he is presented as offering an open challenge to the "best of the Argives" (*Il.* 3.19) as Trojans and Greeks faced each other before the gates of Troy. However, when his challenge is answered by Menelaus, Paris, fearful, retreats back to the "throng of his comrades" (3.33) whereupon Hector berates him. Paris's next speech event is in response to Hector, but his speech is private and spoken only to Hector. In this speech Paris suggests that he and Menelaus meet in single combat for Helen and her dowry. Finally, in his last speech act, when Paris had been whisked back to his chambers from the battlefield by Aphrodite, he must respond to Helen's rebukes of cowardness against him. However, Paris brushes off such criticisms and instead speaks of his passion and desire that they be "bedded together in love" (3.441). In the three speech acts of Paris in book 3, he does not speak authoritatively to Greek and Trojan warriors, that is publicly and as a son of king; instead his words are boastful, mollifying, quiet, and private—the speech acts of a commoner, woman, child, or even slave. The failure of Paris's (masculinity and therefore proper humanity) prowess can be seen in his speech acts which signify Paris as weak, empty, ephemeral and ineffectual. Menelaus, however, demonstrates his command of speech and his position as a properly masculine human when he publicly calls Paris out, and authoritatively reprimands Zeus for allowing his sword to miss its mark preventing him from killing Paris (3.365–368).

In the *Iliad* and *Odyssey* non-human animals occupy an ontological space apart from human animals even if they both daily share the same space. The different ontological spaces for human and non-human animals are constituted in part in the *Iliad* and *Odyssey* through the criteria of shared flesh or kinship and speech.[18] The boundary between non-human and human animals is an important one in the Homeric tales since it metaphorically establishes other kinds of separation within the text, for example, proper speech is only given to men by Homer. Heath has argued that although the texts are not interested in differentiating non-human and human animals per se, they are interested in establishing that proper speech, called authoritative speech, followed by proper action, belongs to adult men, and not women, children, the low-born and slaves. Although some of these "lesser beings" are given lines in the texts, their speech does not carry authority as they do not have command of human, read authoritative, speech (Heath 2005, 77). Like non-human animals, then, these "not-properly-human" people are "other" to the normative human, that is proper men, and are marked as thus by their lack of authoritative speech. These others are signified as other by this lack, a lack inherent to non-human animals the latter of whom act as a binary by which to deauthorize the other locating them, like non-human animals, as the tools of properly masculine humans.

Pain, Bodies, and Boundaries in the Homeric Epics

The Greek word for pain, ποινή or *poinê*, does not appear with any frequency in either the *Iliad* or *Odyssey*. Indeed, according to Liddell and Scott (1968), *poinê* appears only twenty times in the *Iliad* and twice in the *Odyssey*. Considering that pain is a central to both stories, pain in the way we understand it, this seems rather odd. However, *poinê* in the context of these texts refers us to blood money, were-guild, fine, price, or penalty paid (Liddell and Scott 1968), quite a different meaning than I am seeking. Even Greek words (and their cognates) such as ἄλγος (*algos*) referring to pain generally and ἀλγέω (*algeô*), to feel bodily pain, to suffer (s.v. Liddell and Scott 1968), do not always engage the flesh of the body in their reference to pain: pain is metaphorical, emotional, or psychological. Another interesting set of terms for pain are τλῆ (*tlê*) and τλάω (*tlaô*) which speak to suffering and undergoing hardship (*tlê*), or to dare (or not) to do something (*tlaô*) (s.v. Liddell and Scott 1968).[19] However, even if at times these terms hint at ritual suffering inflicted on the body, for example in the characters of Ares when he is said to have endured/suffered, τλῆ, for thirteen months bound in a "brazen jar" (*Il*. 5.385) or Achilles in his fast prior to Patroclus's funeral (*Il*., 19.305–308), the body in its fleshiness tends to be absent. There are of course other terms for pain in the Homeric texts, but these refer more often to states of mind or visitation of sorrows such as δύη (*duê*) and πῆμα (*pêma*) referring to misery and anguish, and misery and calamity (s.v. Liddell and Scott 1968) or μόγις (*mogis*), meaning toil and pain and referring to difficulty (for example, see *Il*. 21.417–418). The tendency of these words and their cognates is to metaphorically engage pain in a textual effort to emphasize or strengthen the event or action described in the text.

If the body is absent in ποινή (*poinê*),[20] ἄλγος (*algos*) and ἀλγέω (*algeô*), τλῆ (*tlê*), τλάω (*tlaô*), δύη (*duê*) and πῆμα (*pêma*) and μόγις (*mogis*), it is present in ὀδύνη (*odunê*) (with a frequency of ten times in the *Iliad* and twice in the *Odyssey*) referring to pain of the body (s.v. Liddell and Scott 1968) making the term useful for the task at hand.[21] Two other terms that speak to pain by referencing groans and sighs are στενάχω (*stenakhô*) and στονόεις (*stonoeis*), the first referring to the voicing of these bodily sounds of pain, and the second to having caused such sounds to occur (s.v. Liddell and Scott 1968). But even here, as with *algos*, they also used to speak of sorrow, lamentation, and sadness (seventeen times in the *Iliad* and nine in the *Odyssey*). They do, however, act on five occasions in the *Iliad* and one in the *Odyssey* as a muted audio register of a body in pain.[22] Both, then, should also be somewhat useful to track the indexical sign of fleshy pain in the Homeric texts.

Deity, non-human animal, hybrid, semi-divine, and human animal all experience pain in the Homeric texts; even the earth metaphorically groans under the weight of the armies when they come together in conflict. In book 5 of the *Iliad*, for example, is the wounding of Aphrodite. In this scene Aeneas has been overcome by the Athena-goaded Diomedes and his death is immanent. His mother Aphrodite, however, steps in and whisks her son from battle. Undeterred, Diomedes pursues Aphrodite and Aeneas wounding her and drawing *ichor* (divine equivalent of blood) from her hand. Dropping her son (whom Apollo helpfully catches), she flees from the battle, and borrowing the chariot of Ares seeks healing from her mother in Olympus (*Il*. 5.334–370). Dione, when healing Aphrodite, speaks to her of other gods who have also suffered pain at the hands of humans, listing Ares, Hera, and Hades (5.370–414). Aphrodite's pain is intense ἀχθομένην ὀδύνῃσι, which A. T. Murray translates as "suffered dreadfully" (5.354). Ares, Hera, and Hades all suffered, τλῆ, (s.v. Liddell and Scott 1968): Ares bound and locked in a "brazen jar"; Hera wounded by the arrow of the son of Amphitryon; and Hades likewise wounded by an arrow. Hera felt pain unbearable (ἀνήκεστον λάβεν ἄλγος), while Hades was given over to pain (βαλὼν ὀδύνῃσιν ἔδωκεν).

Although certainly the deities are separate from humans in Homer's *Iliad*, "a different nation ... [with] a language of their own, [and] their own kind of food ..." (Sissa and Detienne 2000, 18), they nonetheless experience the fullness of human existence (excluding old age and disease) and indeed appear to have the greater share. This greater share can be seen in the amplification of events such as pain, rage, etc. expressed by deity and then visited on the environment in response to their pain.[23] For example, enraged and offended on behalf of his priest Chryses (amplification of the event), Apollo (a powerful if third generation deity) "strode, angry at heart, with his bow and covered quiver on his shoulders ... his coming was like the night ... the mules he attacked first ... but then on men themselves he let fly his stinging arrows ..." (impact on environment) (*Il* 1.44–47). The outcome of Apollo's anger (χωόμενος) was pestilence and death for human and non-human animals alike among the Greek ships until he was mollified by the return of Chryseis, daughter of his priest and the hecatomb offered to him by the Greeks.

The pain of deities is represented as larger than life in the *Iliad* and this is not surprising considering that Greek deities are represented as larger than life. In instances, however, where deities are seen to succumb to pain, they are represented as in a place or situation they should not be or are weak and cowardly. When Aphrodite is wounded by Diomedes, for example, he shouts that she has no place on the battlefield being but a deceiver of "weakling women" (γυναῖκας ἀνάλκιδας). When Ares is wounded he "bellows" (ἔβραχε—*ebrakhe*, rattle, clash, ring) and flees to Olympus seeking retribution from his father Zeus for this insult against him. But Zeus instead thunders, "'Sit not by me and whine, you renegade'" (*Il.* 5.889). So even as deities' pain, anger, love and so forth are writ large, it appears that the overt expression of pain by deities in the *Iliad* is used to register a failing: in the case of Ares, or, as in the wounding of Aphrodite out of place on the battlefield, both operated out of their proper ken and therefore subject to the vicissitudes of existence. Pain is a central component of battle and those who enter the field best be prepared to deal with it.

In the narrative environment of the Homeric texts, a deity's rage, grief and pain are very much amplified and this kind of amplification is also seen among the human characters marked as extraordinary such as the figure of the heroic warrior. The wrath (μῆνιν) of Achilles, the ultimate warrior of

Greek mythology, for example, is a wrath markedly greater in its effect, carried through the entirety of the text as it is, than the anger of Thersites, who is jeered, shamed, and beaten for his anger in book 2 of the *Iliad* (2.211–277). And if rage is important in the *Iliad*, so too is pain, but the kind of pain that is presented is often emotional pain, mental anguish, deep shame, loss, misery, and grief. This kind of pain is central to the telling of the Homeric epics, but the signification of bodily pain, pain in the flesh of the human animal, is negligible to the point of absence, and when it is overtly expressed, that is by more than a "grunt" or "groan" (στενάχω *stenakhô*) and στονόεις (*stonoeis*), it signifies the character "problematic" lacking, as the character does, the appropriate attributes that mark "him" as properly masculine. For example, when Aeneas is wounded by Diomedes:

> With this [a huge stone] he struck Aeneas on the hip, where the thigh turns in the hip joint-the cup, men call it-and crushed the cup, and in addition broke both sinews, and the jagged stone tore the skin away. Then the warrior fell on his knees and remained there, and with his stout hand he leaned on the earth; and dark night enfolded his eyes.
>
> (*Iliad* 5.297–310)

Aeneas is represented as severely and painfully wounded, but no expression of pain is provided. Marking his heroic status is his quick return to battle having been healed by Leto and Artemis (*Il.* 5.512). Another instance of a silent death lacking reference to pain is the sad narrative of Amarynceus. We read he met his fate when first his right leg near the ankle was crushed with a thrown stone and then when Perios, "dealt him a wound with a thrust of his spear beside the navel; and out on to the ground gushed his bowels, and darkness enfolded his eyes" (*Il.* 4.517–526). As with Aeneas, then, when injury is done to his flesh no scream of anguish or desperate cry of pain is made to escape Amarynceus's lips.

These examples of the passing over of fleshy pain are repeated throughout the *Iliad* and *Odyssey* with heroes at best emitting groans or sighs. The apparent absence of pain is striking and is suggestive of one or several things. It could suggest to the reader a "taken-for-granted" of the normativity of pain in war, so much so that warriors' pain is unremarked and unremarkable. Pain and its absence could be the register for the properly masculine warrior insofar as not to acknowledge pain and to do so, beyond a "grunt or groan," is to be unmanned and thus to fail as a hero. Finally, the absence of pain could also mean that the register for pain in the Homeric texts is different from that of the modern reader's and registers of pain.

The first suggestion, that pain is so normative to human life that its textual signification is as unnecessary to register as urination and defecation, is questionable in light of how deities' pain is registered and indeed contributes to the telling of the story and more so to the aggrandizement of the heroic figure, such as Diomedes. Compare, for example, how Ares when wounded bellows as "loud as nine thousand warriors or ten thousand cry in battle ..." (*Il.* 5.859-861) to Diomedes wounding which he shrugs off (*Il.* 11.399-400). If pain was normative and unnecessary to remark on, then one might infer that the pain of deities should also go unremarked, and yet the pain of Ares and Aphrodite is writ large and used to signify a problem with the characters as suggested above. It would appear, then, that pain has a rhetorical function (Aphrodite and Ares) in the texts, as much as its absence (Aeneas and Amarynceus) does.

The second suggestion that the endurance of pain as the signification of a proper heroic masculinity (as with authoritative speech), is eminently viable since warriors who succumb to pain (and death) are seen as having failed the test and in this failure are neither properly masculine nor heroic. As seen with Ares, the unrestricted and overt response to pain, or, as in the case of Paris (*Il.*3.30-37), the obvious avoidance to risk pain and death, register as lack and signals then a failure. If, then, overt responses to pain and/or its avoidance marks failure, the willingness to risk and silently endure pain signify as success and acts as a positive register for proper masculinity.

For example, in book 19 of the *Odyssey*, we are given a tale of Odysseus's wounding during a boar hunt. J. C. B. Petropoulos (2011, 105-120) argues convincingly that Odyssey's trip to see his maternal grandfather in Parnassos references a rite of passage: that of Odysseus's coming of age as a man and warrior. Following the completion of the rite he claimed his inheritance promised to him by his maternal grandfather at his naming ceremony (*Od.* 19.399-412). In the tale of Odysseus's wounding by a wild boar (the same kind of non-human animal that gored the young lover of Aphrodite, Adonis) the tusk of the boar enters above his knee[24] but did not strike the bone. Odysseus's wound was tended "skillfully" and "the black blood checked with a charm" (19.56-57), while Odysseus remained steadfastly silent enduring the pain of the wound and ministrations that followed. The young Odysseus, having endured the pain and survived his wounding, is feasted, gifted and returned home a properly masculine male ready to "give the first performance of his 'personal experience narrative' (or 'personal legend')" (Petropoulos 2011, 120).[25] In this vignette, the absence of an overt response to pain is one of the significations of Odyssesus's having crossed the threshold from youth (*ephebe*) just sprouting a beard to adult man; a properly masculine male who is able to take his appropriate place in the community (ibid., 117-120).

The absence of pain is one positive signification of pain, but another is a begrudging acknowledgement of pain, and this too is used as a further register of a properly masculine warrior's overt ability to endure pain beyond what non-heroic men are able to do. In book 11 of the *Iliad*, for example, Agamemnon, Diomedes and Odysseus, successful heroes of the Achaeans, are each wounded in succession, and each shrugs off the wound, even as the wound requires that they withdraw, briefly, from the intensity of the battle. Agamemnon is the first to be wounded, but he ignores the wound and continues fighting until the blood from his wound dries and "sharp pangs" (ὀξεῖ' ὀδύναι), like the pain of women's childbirth, seize him and force him to retreat from battle (*Il.* 11.248-283). Diomedes, also in the thick of the struggle, is then struck in the foot by Paris's arrow, and, taunted by Paris, jeers back that Paris lacks proper masculinity since he refuses to fight him in a "trial of ... man to man in armour." And, even as he threatens Paris, Diomedes, a properly masculine warrior, unlike Paris, a failed warrior who like an *ephebe* carries a bow, scoffs at his wound: "I care not for it, any more than if a woman had struck me, or a witless child, for blunt is the dart of one who is a weakling and a nobody" (11.384-389). Taking refuge behind Odysseus, Diomedes withdraws the arrow and "a painful pang shot through his flesh" (ὀδύνη δὲ διὰ χροὸς ἦλθ' ἀλεγεινή) bringing about his temporary withdrawal from battle (11.398).

Finally, Odysseus, as much a warrior as Agamemnon and Diomedes, is wounded with a spear in the side, but he too makes little of the wound as he turns on his attacker and kills him (*Il.* 11.439-445). Like both Agamemnon and Diomedes, Odysseus too must withdraw from battle due to his wound, but their withdrawal from battle is brief as they quickly heal from their wounds, being proper warriors. As heroic warriors, properly masculine and fully human, the hero kings Agamemnon, Diomedes and Odysseus endure and suffer, and but they are never overcome by pain of body since to succumbing to pain signifies failed warrior.

In book 16 of the *Iliad*, this necessity not to be overtaken by pain is made explicit when Galucus, wounded by an arrow and unable to assist the dying Sarpedon, prays to Apollo for help:

> I have this terrible wound, and my arm is shot through with sharp pangs, nor can the blood be dried; and my shoulder is made heavy with the wound, and I cannot hold my spear firmly, nor go and fight with the foe ... but you my lord, at least heal me of this terrible wound, and lull my pains (ὀδύνας) ...
> (*Iliad* 16.515-524)

Sarpedon dying, requests that Glaucus retrieve his body and armor and if

Glaucus should fail in this request, then Sarpedon promises "for to you even in time to come shall I be a rebuke and a cause of shame all your days continually ..." (16.498–500). Faced with possible shame, potentially unmanned by his wound, and therefore questionably masculine, Glaucus calls on Apollo, tutelary deity of *ephebes* (Graf 2009, 103–113), young males crossing over the threshold from youth to adulthood, to redress the situation and allow him to reclaim his masculinity so that he could secure Sarpedon's body and armour. Pain, then, when threatening to overtake a warrior, signifies a potential failure of masculinity unless the situation is remedied and the warrior can then properly engage in combat. When warriors withdraw from the front line of combat to mix among the throng of soldiers, others jeer or scold them such as Hector did to Paris. Avoiding the risk of pain means unwillingness to endure and overcome pain indicating the potential warrior is not properly masculine (and womanly or childishly) and therefore not an adult male (and therefore of the *ephebes*).[26]

Finally, some might infer that the texts may have another kind of register for pain, and rather than a speaking to suffering that comes from the inside to spill outside through the mouth as in, for example: "the pain ripped out from her throat in an anguished screamed" or "he wept and cried as the pain tore through him," in the Homeric texts the register for pain may be signified in the description of the wound itself. The modern textual literary register for pain is found in the words and sounds that provide access to the "inner" world of the suffering "self" in the text. This idea of an "inner world" and suffering self is taken to be the truth of pain in the modern Eurowestern context, and this way of thinking about pain has been shaped by the concept of a soul, something found only later in the classical context, and then subsequently in early Christianities (among other systems of belief and practice).[27]

The belief in an "inner self," be it a soul, a self, or even multiple selves contained by and in the fleshy body, continues to dominant current understandings of the body and self (Hall 2000). In Homeric texts, however, there is no distinguishing between an inside and an outside: there are words, deeds, and acts which culminate in what Petropoulos (2011, 120) calls the "personal legend," composed of multiple narratives that together create a story that constructs the "self." In part, then, the texts lack a representation of an "inner self" whereby pain can flow from the inside to the outside, and instead the reader is presented with vivid and detailed descriptions of bodily damage that act as literary registers of pain: "and the helmet and the horsehair crest was split about the spear point ... and the brain all mingled with blood spurted out from the wound along the socket of the spear" (*Il.* 17.295–298).

The Homeric visual cues of bodies torn, crushed, and bloodied may well be the textual site where pain is spoken. Here the visual register, that is torn, ripped flesh, gapping and bloody holes in bellies, heads, and chests, allows the reader to measure the pain the hero endures and must overcome silently if he is to hold his warrior status, requiring as it does that he not succumb to pain. Through description and visual registers for pain, the reader can more readily empathize with, even as they recognize the properly adult, masculine, heroic warrior. Equally, the succumbing to pain or the unwillingness to endure pain acts to register a character's unmanning or having lacked proper heroic masculinity from the outset: he has failed as a hero.

This use of the indexical sign, pain, as a means to mark failure and therefore lack is evident throughout the text, but nicely exemplified in such scenes as the death of Dolon found in book 10 of the *Iliad*, wherein Dolon, hunted by Odysseus and Diomedes, shrieks and then falls into the dust dead (*Il.* 10.363), and in the scene of Achaean and Trojan confrontation in front of the walls of Troy wherein Paris must be shamed by Hector before he will face Menelaus in single combat. To endure pain is the role of the properly masculine warrior and to signify this endurance are the graphic visualizations of pain that dominant the narrative of the *Iliad*.

When it comes to pain and non-human animals, as with deities and human animals, the Homeric texts use pain to signify in particular ways. Some animals at times are represented as having the capacity to experience pain, and therefore appear to share this faculty with humans and deities. For example, we read of an eagle speeding away with a sharp or piercing cry (κλάγξας klagxas) when stung with pain (ἀλγήσας ὀδύνῃσι) by the snake it held in its talons (*Il.*12.205-206). Pain is registered by the non-human animal, but the eagle is a *wild* animal rather than the domestic non-human animal, and it is the latter whose pain is typically unremarked upon in the text. That said, there is one domestic non-human animal whose pain is signified and therefore registered: the horse, a non-human animal that has a higher status than other domestic animals such as oxen, mules, or sheep, especially when it comes to war and hunting. Even so, when horses, away from the field of war or the paths of the hunt, like other domestic animals, are marked for sacrifice, food, or labor their pain is absent or minimally registered in the texts.

The most obvious textual events where pain goes unregistered but at the same time is significant to its performance, is sacrifice[28]: "they first drew back the victims' heads, and cut their throats, and flayed them ..." (*Il.* 2.423); "four horses with high arched necks he cast swiftly on the pyre ... nine dogs ... of these Achilles cut the throats of two, and cast them on the pyre" (*Il.* 23.171-174); or with minimal comment "[h]e spake, and cut the lambs' throats with the pitiless bronze; and laid them down upon the ground gasping and failing of breath, for the bronze had robbed them of their strength" (Il. 3.292-3).[29] Animals led to the sacrifice are not represented as bellowing and crying in pain or even struggling to flee their captors (e.g., Od 11.30-34). Some might conjecture that this should come as no surprise in light of the ancient context wherein there was considerable contact, and therefore general ease, between domestic animals and humans and this ease was reflected in the Homeric texts. Furthermore, one might argue, the kind of blow dealt to the sacrificial animal and the cutting of its throat would prevent crying out, while the rapid bleeding from such a wound would prevent struggle. In another vein, one might argue that the absence of a register for domestic, non-human animal pain could suggest non-human animal pain is not thought, in other words there is a blindness to it, an ignorance that serves the social body at large.

As arguments against these readings for the absence of non-human animal pain, in the first instance it would only be during preparation to the sacrifice that the animal would acquiesce, but in those few seconds when the knife first cuts the throat, struggle and pain must necessarily be present, and therefore for it to be elided in the texts suggests that there is something at stake in the absence of the sign of pain. The second conjecture, that non-human animal pain is not "thought" in the texts, is also unsatisfying since non-human animal pain is registered with some animals and at different times in the *Iliad* as evidenced with the eagle and the horse.

In the quotidian of the texts, domestic, non-human animals are represented as tools and possessions owned by human animals. This understanding of non-human animals is nicely evidenced during the funeral games of Patroclus wherein horses and mules (along with captured women) are listed among the prizes to be given out by Achilles (*Il.* 23.262-270). In the texts non-human animals are used for food (goats, sheep, bovines, pigs) (see *Il.* 3.25) and necessities such as cloth, shields, and bow strings (oxen) (see *Il.* 17.389-395 in particular), for hunting and livestock management (dogs) (see *Il.* 8.338-339; 9.545; 10.183; 12.303; 18.578), transportation (horses and oxen), and growing food (mules and oxen), and in this, then, live side-by-side with human animals. Therefore, living together as closely as they did suggests the pain of domestic animals registers in its absence.

If explicit reference to bodily pain is absent, however, the laborious effort of non-human animals speaking to strain is registered. Read in book 17 of the *Iliad*, for example, mules are said to strive with great effort and strength so that their hearts (θυμὸς) are "distressed (τείρεθ') (*teireth*) with weariness and sweat ..." (744-745), but pain, bodily pain, linked to such effort is not registered and at best can only be inferred (see also *Il.* 23.121-122, and with reference to oxen see *Il.* 13.703-705).

If in sacrifice non-human animal pain is absent in both the *Iliad* and *Odyssey*, suggesting a willingness on the part of sacrifice, something that was might have been central to later Greek and Roman animal sacrifice (the *hupokupein*), and in labor their enduring effort is registered but certainly not as pain, while warfare moves one non-human animal, the horse, into the conceptual space of the human animal to share some of the warrior's story. Domestic, non-human animal pain with relation to the war horse makes apparent the absence of a register for other non-human animals. In the Homeric texts, like many war epics ancient and modern,[30] it is the war horse[31] that is made to register the indexical sign of pain.

Horses appear in the catalogue of ships, "of the horses best by far were the mares of the sons of Pheres ... Apollo of the silver bow reared Pereia, both of them mares, bringing with them the panic of war" (*Il.* 2.763-767). Achilles's horse speaks to him, and horses are represented as part of the warrior's accoutrements of war affiliated as they are with the chariot. The deities, Zeus (*Il.* 8.41-46), Hera (*Il.* 4.27), Hera and Athena (*Il.* 8.374-382), Ares (*Il.* 5.851), and Poseidon (*Il.* 13.32-38) all have horses and chariots, and although Iris and Aphrodite (along with Hephaestos, Apollo, and Artemis) are not represented in chariots drawn by horses, they are still capable of handling horses and driving chariots, demonstrated at least when they borrow Ares's chariot (*Il.* 5.363-366). Horses with chariots in tow (*Il.* 23.192 ff.) participate in dirges (*Il.* 23.10-15) and funeral (*Il.* 23.128-139), and marriage (*Od.* 4.1-19) processions. Furthermore, horses, like heroes have their own lineages and narratives (*Il.* 2.763-767; 263-269) and like warriors they are honored (*Il.* 8.184-190). In warfare horses take battle orders (*Il.* 16. 684), face evil toil and death (*Il.* 17.400; 21.520-521), deliver death (*Il.* 5.587), and weep over the dead (*Il.* 17.425-455). Horses are valuable and therefore stolen (*Il.* 5.640-643; *Od.* 21.15-30), given as gifts (*Il.* 9.121-124; 10.305-306; *Od.* 4.589-592), or sacrificed (*Il.* 21.130-132; 23.170-172), and are used to mark a warrior's capacity (*Il.* 11.127-130) or lack therein, as with Dolon who, in book 10 of the *Iliad*, took up his bow, and putting on the skin of a wolf and a ferret-skin cap sought to spy on the Achaeans in order that he may claim the chariot and horses of Achilles should the Trojans prove successful in the war (*Il.* 11.321-323). When Odysseus surmises the reward that drove Dolon to spy on the Achaeans, he comments with a smile that these horses were well beyond Dolon's capacity to master or drive (*Il.* 10.400-404).[32] And, not be forgotten, it was a giant wooden horse that allow the Achaeans to bring about the defeat of the horse-taming Trojans (*Od.* 8.487-488).

It is clear from the above, and particularly in light of some horses (like some warriors) having personal identity narratives attached to their names, that there was much more to the horse than there was to the ox, the mule, the goat, the sheep, and even the dog, which often, like the horse, carried a different status in the heroic narratives. Indeed, in some ways the horse as companion animal seen in the *Iliad* is replace by the dog as companion animal in the *Odyssey* evidenced by Telemachos's turning back Menelaus's gift of horses (*Od.* 4.595–608); in Odysseus's horselessness, and in the loyal hound Argus's recognition of Odysseus (*Od.* 17.290–327).

In the *Iliad*, the horse and the warrior are intimately tied together, and as one faces war, so too does the other. The catalogue of ships in book 2 lists horses along with men and chariots making apparent the importance of the horse to the warriors of *Iliad*, albeit this is significantly less the case for the Odyssey.[33] In book 2 (386) of the *Iliad*, for example, men see to their horses in preparation for battle, and in books 13 (683–684) and 15 (352–355) horses and men come together in the crush of battle bound in "furious fight." As a text of warfare, the narrative of the war horse, like that of the warrior, plays a significant role in the text, and it is unsurprising that, unlike other non-human animals, some horses can share metaphorical kinship with the human animal.

Patroclus's horse, Pedasus, fulfills the role of war horse in the *Iliad* and his pain is made to register. In book 16 Patroclus engaged in the battle around the Achaean ships and the spear of Sarpedon, aimed at Patroclus, struck Pedasus his horse "on the right shoulder; and the horse shrieked (bellowed) (ἔβραχε) as it gasped out its life, and down it fell in the dust with a moan (κὰδ δ' ἔπεσ' ἐν κονίῃσι μακών), and its spirit flew from it" (ἀπὸ δ' ἔπτατο θυμός) (*Il.* 16.465–469).[34] The phrase κὰδ δ' ἔπεσ' ἐν κονίῃσι μακών (*kad d' epes' en koniêsi makôn*) "fell shrieking to earth" spoken of a wounded horse, stag, or boar" is formulaic and used to speak of the death of horses and wild animals in war or the hunt (s.v Liddell and Scott 1968), however the term is twice applied with reference to questionably masculine men, something I return to below.

The figure of the horse, then, unlike other domesticated non-human animals, had achieved a particular status in the text of the *Iliad* able, as some few among them are, to acquire immortality, brief speech, comprehension of speech, honor, and heroic narratives attached to their names. With this kind of distinction among non-human animals, it is not surprising that horses are represented in the *Iliad* as suffering pain when wounded. Similar to the wounding of Pedasus, is the wounding of Nestor of Gerenia's horse: "So, stung with agony the horse leapt on high as the arrow sank into his brain, and he threw into confusion horses and car as he writhed upon the bronze. (*Il.* 8.85–86). Horses in warfare carry a different status; they are fellow combatants and in some sense fellow warriors, requiring bravery since they too faced death (*Il.* 21.520–521). When figured as "fellow warriors" this enhanced status was operative, but when the horse is positioned as sacrifice or laboring, the horse, like other non-human animals, is given no pain in the text. The absence of the sign of pain read through a poststructural lens represents a negative register that then points to how pain, although shared by all, belongs properly only to some; deities, humans, wild animals, and the war horse.

Pain and its Significations in the Homeric Texts

Deities, humans, and non-human animals are separate signs, and although the borders between are porous at times, this porousness is marked as extraordinary and typically brings tragedy: when Xanthas is given speech by Hera, he foretells the latter's death. There are sharp boundaries between the three signs, but even as the boundaries are there, they are crossed repeatedly while pain (along with kinship and speech) acts as the indexical sign, a rhetoric of the flesh, that marks proper boundaries and even proper ways of being. Pain, and its absence, marks those who fall outside or inside, and marks and secures the boundaries between deity, human, and non-human animals.

This marking of boundaries is nicely registered in the phrase "fell shrieking to earth" (κὰδ δ' ἔπεσ ἐν κονίῃσι μακών) (μακών—bleat, moan, scream, shriek), which is used three times in the *Iliad* and four times in the *Odyssey*, and typically applied to non-human animal pain and death, but on two occasions it is applied to humans in the Homeric texts. In terms of non-human animals, in the *Odyssey* the phrase "feel shrieking to the earth" is used to refer to a stag's death (10.163) and to the death of a boar (19.454), while in book 9 only μακών is used and applied to the bleating sound ewes make when needing to be milked. In the *Iliad* book 16 the phrase is used to represent the horse Pedasus's death, while μακών is used in book 9 to refer to the sound of the Trojans preparing for battle (439). In all but two instances of its use in both texts, *makôn*, ewes bleating with full udders, and *kad d' epes' en koniêsi makôn*, felling shrieking to the earth, explicitly act as registers of non-human animal distress.

However, even as the term and phrase register non-human animal distress, when applied to a Trojan warrior or braggart beggar of the *Odyssey*, they move the subject from the normative human, in this instance properly masculine adult male, to the space of the non-human animal and therefore no longer belonging to the imaginary community of Homeric warriors. In book 10 of the *Iliad* the Trojan warrior Dolon, likened to a hunted animal, runs shrieking μεμηκώς (*memêkôs*) before the dogs as he is pursued by Odysseus and Diomedes (363). Dolon, caped with wolf skin and capped with ferret fur, had furtively approached the Achaean encampment when he was surprised by Diomedes and Odysseus who had quietly laid among the dead. Fleeing, Diomedes stops him with a spear throw and Dolon is "seized with terror, stammering and pale with fear, and the chattering of his teeth was heard through his lips" (*Il.* 10.374–377). Dolon pleads for his life, betrays the Trojans, and is then beheaded by Diomedes. Odysseus, party to the event, takes Dolon's wolf pelt and ferret cap (along with bow and arrows) and later "places the blood-stained spoils of Dolon [on the stern of his ship] until they should prepare a sacred offering to Athene" (*Il.* 10.570): Interestingly Dolon's animal garb is what Odysseus thinks to sacrifice to Athena along with his spear and bow signifying Dolon's death as a sacrifice.

Ἀκών (*akôn*) and its application to non-human animals in particular, is nicely suggestive of how pain—its presence and absence—is able to act as a register that marks a boundary between non-human animals and human animals. When hunted or wounded in war they are made to scream, shriek, and tremble when wounded, marking their incapacity to endure. This lack in the non-human animal is the rhetorical device by which to signify problematic masculinity for those who, like non-human animals, are unable to endure pain. An internal boundary is generated using non-human animal pain to mark those who are improperly male and masculine. For example, like Dolon, the "public beggar" Arnaeus, "known as Irus by the young men,"[35] foolishly tries to drive the disguised Odysseus from the threshold of Penelope's door and is subsequently challenged to a wrestling match by Odysseus. Irus, originally filled with bravado, trembles, and shakes when faced with the shapely, stout thighs and mighty chest and arms of Odysseus. Irus must be led to the ring where he is severely wounded and falls to the "dust with a moan." Likened to the wounding and killing of an animal (stag or boar), Irus is unmanned and publicly shamed by Odysseus, while his bodily pain is used to send a message to the suitors of Penelope (*Od.* 18.1–107). Irus attempts what he is incapable of doing: demonstrating his lack of proper human adult masculinity.

The indexical sign of pain, its absence and presence that are either resisted or yielded to, is a means by which to speak about the ontology of deities, humans and non-human animals and mark the boundaries between. Pain, and its absence, is a register that marks a similarity between all three kinds, but equally it is a register that separates one from the other so that three kinds are definable as distinct. In the Homeric texts, deities experience pain as humans do and one non-human domestic animal the horse, at least when they are not sacrificed: in sacrifice their pain has no place in the text. Deities like humans when overcome by pain are marked as not properly masculine and therefore ill-placed (Aphrodite) or ill-equipped (Ares) to deal with the work of warriors. And although the war horse is given his own heroic tale, at least in terms of the field of battle, and for a moment shares in the gifts of the human animal—if he does not, of course, succumb to pain and fear (*Il.* 6.37–41; 12.50–54). But even as one non-human animal registers pain, when it comes to sacrifice and labor—serving as the tools of the human animals, the pain of non-human animals is absent and it is this absence of pain that reinforces the boundary between the non-human animal, the human animal and deity(ies). Humans and deities endure and overcome pain, and therefore pain acts as a register of their proper being, while those who fall prey to pain (and death) signify failure as they have been overcome by the task at hand. Equally, in this heroic play of masculinity and pain, the overt response to pain by deity, warrior or war horse marks the character as succumbing to pain and therefore signifying as weak. Sacrificial and laboring animals, including the horse, however, lack a register of pain and it is this absence that reveals the assumptions of the Homeric texts that takes for granted a vast gulf that separates non-human animals from human animals. Furthermore, the text uses the sign of non-human animal to rhetorically mark kinds of people as problematic and/or non-normative.

The Mayan Popol Vuh

The Mayan alphabetic *Popol Vuh* or Book of Council (also Book of the People) of the K'iche' Maya of Guatemala, was written down in the sixteenth century during the period of initial Spanish colonization in the town of K'iche' (Tedlock 1996, 25). If the alphabetic text of *Popol Vuh* is dated to the sixteenth century CE, however, the myth can be dated hieroglyphically to the post-Classic period (1200–1521 CE) (Joyce 2000, 77), evidenced from Temple XIX at Palanque dated to the late Classic period (550–850 CE) (Stewart 2005), and Maya lowland pottery representations of the themes in the *Popol Vuh* seen in the Classic period (250 CE–1000 CE) (Tedlock 2010, 301). The authors of the *Popol Vuh* write, "We shall write about this now amid the preaching of God in Christendom now. We shall bring it out because there is no longer/ a place to see it, a council book ..." (Tedlock 1996, 63). When the Spanish colonizers arrived, they quickly began to destroy the books of the Maya and declare the Mayan script to be non-writing and the works of the devil. In the face of this, the Maya concealed their written works. The *Popol Vuh* next surfaces in the small town of Chuvila (Santo Tomás Chichicasteango) and it is here in the early eighteenth century that the local parish priest Francisco Ximénez saw and then copied the document. His translation was kept by the Dominicans until the library of the University of San Carlos in Guatemala City acquired it in the mid-nineteenth century (Tedlock 1996, 27; Christenson 2007, 39).

Toward the end of the nineteenth century, copies and translations of the document began to appear, while the Ximénez copy was in Newberry Library (Chicago) by 1911 (Tedlock 1996, 27). Drawing on updated and corrected work on the manuscript, discussions with scholars and linguists, art and architecture, newly translated hieroglyphs, and discussions with living K'iche' Maya mother-fathers and day keepers, Dennis Tedlock and Allen Christenson developed their translations of the *Popol Vuh*.

Popol Vuh Kinship and Speech

The *Popol Vuh* of the K'iche' Maya of Guatemala, like the ancient Homeric texts, constructs a boundary between the non-human and human animal, and to do so the concepts of kinship and speech are also significant for marking boundaries, as they were in the Homeric texts. Equally, the indexical sign, pain, plays a similar rhetorical function in the *Popol Vuh* as it signifies a failure or a debacle, whereas its absence, as in the Homeric texts, signifies a success or a triumph. The *Popol Vuh*, however, is not concerned with demarcating the weak from the strong based on an ideology of warrior masculinity; rather, the presence and absence of the indexical sign of pain marks a hierarchy of beings and peoples, some of whom will serve and be served, be eaten and eat, and act as sacrifices or sacrificers to the deities.

The text of the K'iche' *Popol Vuh* tells the story of the emergence of deities, creation, and beings mapping out the boundaries of existence. This myth, like any creation myth, was foundational to the K'iche' Maya and their social formations and interaction with the local flora and fauna; although certainly interpretation and ideological use of the *Popol Vuh* differs according to different historical periods and cultural, political, social, and/or economic needs.[36] In the creation myth of the *Popol Vuh* several efforts are required to bring human animals into existence. The first effort to create the "human design," and the second act of creation, brought non-human animals into existence directly after land and water were brought into existence. Both the first and second acts of creation are done with *the thoughts and words* of the deities Hurricane, Newborn Thunderbolt, Sudden Thunderbolt, Heart of Sky, Heart of Earth, Maker, Modeler, Bearer, Begetter. Once created, non-human animals are made guardians of the forests and requested by the deities to "speak, pray to us, keep our days" (Tedlock 1996, 67). But bird, deer, serpent, and puma (undomesticated) are unable to comply with this request and so they are "brought low" and although named the "guardians of forests and bushes," and therefore primal beings, they must accept their service to the anticipated human design (ibid., 68).

The deities continue their efforts to find the right time and means to create proper beings who can pray and keep the ritual days and next the mud people and then the manikins are created, both of which are failed acts of creation, like non-human animals, and are subsequently destroyed (the myth explains that a few of the manikins survived and became the monkeys of the forest as well as dwell in Xbalba, the underworld of the *Popol Vuh*). Humans do not arrive on the scene until the fifth act of creation wherein the makers, modelers, Bearer Xpiyacoc and Begetter Xmucane use staple foods, located by fox, coyote, parrot and crow on Good Mountain, to create the four mother-fathers: Xmucane grinds the "yellow corn, white corn alone for the flesh, food alone for the human legs and arms, for our first fathers, the four human works" (Tedlock 1996, 146).

Significantly, in the acts of creation found in the *Popol Vuh*, the opportunity for kinship or a shared genealogy between human and non-human animals is made impossible and indeed marked boundaries are established so that distinct kinds are created. The two groups, non-human and human animals, are distinct kinds in that they are separated by time and space both having come into being in separate events of creation; non-human animals in the second and human animals in the fifth. The gulf of time and space between these two creation events ensures that kinship between human and non-human animals cannot be imagined.

Of equal importance in the creative events of the narrative are the two kinds of activity used to create non-human and human animals. In the act of the creation of non-human animals, thought and word, as with the creation of earth and water, were used: "Then were conceived the animals of the mountains, the guardians of the forest, and all that populate the mountains—the deer and the birds, the puma and the jaguar, the serpent and the rattlesnake, the pit viper and the guardian of the bushes" (Christenson 2004, l. 274–276). However, when creating the human design, the bearer and begetter, Xmucane and Xpiyacoc, use material derived from the first act of creation, maize, that had been supplied by non-human animals. In the myth, Xmucane and Xpiyacoc have been informed about yellow and white corn growing on Good Mountain by fox, coyote, parrot, and crow. They gather the maize and Xmucane, the bearer and midwife, grinds the corn nine times and from it came "the human legs and arms, for our first fathers, the four human works" (Tedlock 1996, 146). Narratively, then, non-human and human animals are further separated by kinds of acts by which they are created, thinking and speaking in the second (and first) act of creation, and "seeking, finding, grinding, rinsing, and speaking in the final act of creation (Tedlock 1996, 145–146; Christenson 2007, 168–171).

The text relays that the newly created humans, the four mother-fathers, are able to do what non-human animals were unable to do: they "speak, pray, and keep the days" and are therefore signified as a successful and complete act of creation. These are the "human works" and even if non-human animals assisted in their creation, there can be no kinship between the two since non-human animals also represent a failed attempt of the human design. Unlike the mud people (second attempt) or manikins (third attempt), however, they were not destroyed and instead are put into the service of those who are able to praise and count the days, the proper human design. In the *Popol Vuh* non-human animals are marked as a failed attempt and this too draws a boundary further establishing an ontological difference between the non-human and human animal. Even as the boundary between human and non-human animals is established, non-human animals are not represented as powerless: They have power in their world of forest and canyon, the primal place of first creation, and their own immeasurable animal power could be beneficial or harmful.

If non-human animals occupy a different category from human animals, and share no kinship, another significant failure that further established this boundary was proper speech, again as in the Homeric texts. The first effort to create the human design brought non-human animals into existence. The creative efforts of the deities were directed toward bringing into existence beings who could speak: to pray and count the days. Sadly, non-human animals could only squawk, chatter and howl when asked to speak and count the days by Maker, Modeler, Bearer, Begetter (Tedlock 1996, 67). Although, these sounds show, as Dennis Tedlock argues, "a potential for articulate speech" (ibid., 230–231), non-human animals cannot speak properly. The deities call out: "Name now our names, praise us. We are your mother, we are your father ... speak, pray to us, keep our days," but "they [did] not hear their speech among the animals. [In light of this lack of realized potential non-human animals must] ... accept your service, just let your flesh be eaten" (ibid., 68).

Speech, then, is another signifier that establishes a boundary between human and non-human animals. As speech or the lack therein figure in the *Popol Vuh*, non-human animals because they lacked articulate speech, even if the potential was there, were cast as a failed creative act and although not destroyed, they are put in the service of human animals. As a failed effort and now in service to the human design, a natural hierarchy is established in *Popol Vuh* whereby human animals use non-human animals as "resources" for labor, food, sport, sacrifice, and sources of power. The ontology of non-human animals in the *Popol Vuh* sets in place a normative understanding of non-human animals as beings completely unrelated to human animals, and furthermore, since they lack speech they are to give themselves over to human animals.

The shaping and the speaking of creations in the *Popol Vuh* sets the human animal at the center of creation, while four of the five acts of creation were efforts to bring about the human design by the deities. In these efforts non-human animals were created and have power that assists both deities and humans, but nonetheless a wide gulf between non-human and human animals remains. Non-human animals cannot speak the language of the deities, they are brought into being as a first effort and separate from subsequent efforts, they are created with thought and word and not substances material and ritual gestures as was the human animal. The distinction made between non-human and human animals related to speech registers negatively insofar as the creative act that produced non-human animals is signified as having gone wrong: because non-human animals cannot speak, they are classified as a failed creation even if they are not destroyed by the deities. Instead, they are allowed to remain in the forest and canyons to serve and to be eaten—to serve because they were failures in creation and to be eaten as they shared no kinship with human animals separated by substance and time. Although non-human animals also signify positively insofar as they, like the land and water, have the power of primordial creation, the power they carry is never used in their own service, but only to serve the deities[37] or humans. Equally, this power marked them as "other" and very different from human animals affirming again their role to serve and to be eaten. The ontological role given to non-human animals is one that is textually set in stone insofar as these differences are established in the existential narrative of the *Popol Vuh*'s cosmogonic myth.

Presence and Absence: Intimations of Pain in the *Popol Vuh*

Pain, *k'ax*[38] in Christenson's (2004) translation of the *Popol Vuh*, unlike kinship and speech, does not appear to reinforce a boundary separating human from non-human animals in any direct way. Instead, pain appears to have another rhetorical function in the *Popol Vuh*. Most of the kinds of beings appear to be subject to pain; that is some deities, and some non-human and human animals. But some is important insofar as those who succumb to pain also fail in their efforts and those who do not succumb succeed in their effort. The indexical sign of pain, then, is important in the myth to signify that a character, act, or event has been compromised and therefore fail. A few examples from the text should suffice to demonstrate this signification of pain, *k'ax*, found the *Popol Vuh*.

In part 1 of the *Popol Vuh*, pain is referenced as that which the manikins and non-human animals experienced when they are either destroyed or brought low. Non-human animals cannot speak and therefore represented a failed act of creation. And although they are not destroyed, as the manikins were, they will now serve and in this service, they will be subject to pain. But they can also administer pain and sent by the deities, the dogs and turkeys (representing domesticated animals) attacked the arrogant manikins who refused to acknowledge the deities, crying "you caused us pain, you ate us, but it is you whom we shall eat." The manikins are also attacked by "[t]he stones, their hearthstones [which] were shooting out, coming right out of the fire, going for their heads," causing the manikins pain (Tedlock 1996, 72).[39] The manikins tried to flee, but most were destroyed except for a few who become monkeys and as such joined the group of non-human animals confirming again the failed state of non-human animals. The transformation of kind, like that effected on the first hero twins' sons, One Monkey and One Artisan, both of whom are transformed into howler monkeys by their nephews Hunahpu and Xbalanque, also reasserted the ontological status of non-human animals in relation to human animals with the first marked as failure and the second as success.

In part 2 of the *Popol Vuh*, when a trace of early dawn appears, the second hero twins Hunahpu and Xbalanque decide that Seven Macaw, with his jeweled eye and tooth, is aggrandizing himself[40] and so must be brought low. Toward this end they devise a plan to ambush Seven Macaw which culminated with Hunahpu losing his arm, but equally Seven Macaw's jaw was injured so much so that he later seeks the ministrations of two boys, the twins in disguise, traveling by his home with a grandmother and grandfather. Because of his pain, insofar as he was completely distracted "[s]ince the lord is getting done in by the pain in his teeth ..." (Tedlock 1996, 80), Seven Macaw makes himself vulnerable to the hero-twins, and is ultimately killed by them. Hunahpu, however, armless for a period of time, is able to retrieve his arm, apparently having suffered no pain either when the arm was torn off or for the duration of its absence. Hunahpu is not represented as having been afflicted with pain thereby signalling his continuing state of success in the *Popol Vuh*.

Part 3 of Tedlock's translation of the *Popol Vuh* tracks the birth and adventures of the hero-twins Hunahpu and Xbalanque, sons of the first set of hero-twins One and Seven Hunahpu who met their end in Xibalba, the underworld realm ruled by One and Seven Death. Ball players, One and Seven Hunahpu had been playing ball at the ball court located on the road to Xibalba. Annoyed and offended, the lords of Xibalba demand the twins play with them the outcome of which was the twins being sacrificed and buried at the place of the ball game sacrifice, while the head of One Hunahpu was placed in a tree by the road. It was the spittle of the head of One Hunahpu that impregnated Blood Moon, daughter of Blood Gatherer a lord of Xbalba. She later gave birth to Hunahpu and Xbalanque, the final set of twins.

In the *Popol Vuh* although One and Seven Hunahpu have managed to traverse the various dangers on the road to Xbalba, they are defeated by One and Seven Death and their failure is made evident in the text when they succumb to pain having sat on the burning bench offered to them by the lords of Xibalba: "So now they were burned on the bench; they really jumped around on the bench now, but they got no relief. They really got up fast, having burned their butts. At this the Xibalbans laughed again ..." (Tedlock 1996, 96). When Hunahpu and Xbalanque make their journey to the underworld, they succeed in all the tests and although they too ultimately meet their death in Xibalba, they are resurrected, defeat the Xibalbans and head to the sky as the sun and moon initiating the beginning of time. Throughout their adventures pain is absent such as when Hunahpu painlessly lost his arm but retrieved it later, and again when his head is removed by the bats of the bat house. Later his brother Xbalanque, with the help of non-human animals, was able to retrieve the head and reattach it on the body of Hunahpu. And, when they return as sorcerers who defeat the Xbalbans, they are able to sacrifice each other with neither overcome by pain.

Part 4 of the *Popol Vuh* narrates the creation of the human design by Xmucane, Xpiyacoc and the primordial non-human animals who found the proper material, white and yellow corn, for the construction of the human design. The primordial aspect of non-human animals the first beings, the mother-fathers, will draw from in order that they may secure human blood and gore to offer to the three deities said to be secured at Tulan: Tohil, Auilix, and Hacauitz. Similar to how the sign of the non-human animal is put into play in Homer's texts, is its use in the demogonic (creation of the group, people, society) myth found in part 4 of the *Popol Vuh*.

Part 4 sets the stage for the necessity of blood offerings to the deity Tohil and who will provide the majority of blood. We read that for Tohil's gift of fire all the tribes, except those belonging to the four great houses of the four mother-fathers, the first humans, are to be subject to "suckling on their sides and under their arms." In other words, they are to be sacrifices giving their heart and blood to Tohil (Tedlock 1996, 155). We read that at the outset that the tribes are numerous and "all alike in dressing with hides. They wore no clothes of the better kind. They were in patches, they were adorned with mere animal hides" (ibid., 152–156). In their non-human animal skins they are marked as lacking ("mere"), but still linked to non-human animals and their power. It may be the tribes had not arrived at their full human potential since they receive their deities at Tulan and only then were they positioned to "speak, pray to us, keep [the] days" (ibid., 67). Furthermore, at Tulan speech is differentiated among the nations so much so that they are unable to understand each other and when the nations approached the four mother-fathers of the K'iche', Jaguar Quitze, Jaguar Night, Not Right Now, Dark Jaguar, to request access to Tohil's fire, their request goes unanswered since their speech was incomprehensible to the four mother-fathers. Once the tribes make their need comprehensible to the mother-fathers of the K'iche', however, the other tribes are told that they must allow themselves to be suckled from the side—that is sacrificed on an altar to Tohil. Throughout part 4 interactions between nations of differing people are played out and the people of the four first mother-fathers (having hid their deities in the Mountains, forests and canyons, the space of non-human animals, those beings who assist, and have access to primordial power) hunted the other nations needing blood and gore offerings for their deities. At first the other nations thought people were being killed by the coyote, puma or jaguar, since the prints and calls of these non-human animals were observed in and around the disappearances. But in time, the Nations realize the K'iche were hunting them in order to "cut them open" before Tohil and Auilix (ibid., 165).

The people of the four-mother fathers lived among and mimicked non-human animals. They drank water and ate the larvae of the yellow jacket, wasp and bee; primal food and drink seemingly marking the primal status of the four mother-fathers and their people. Initially the deities are given resin, blood of the deer and bird, and stitches (blood) from the ear and elbow (penis) of each of the four mother-fathers. But, as promised at Tulan, the nations are to be suckled from their sides by the "penitents" or bloodletters (Christenson 2004, 196) and "sacrificers" (Tedlock 1996, 165) and their blood and gore given over to Tohil, Auilix, and Hacauitz. Coming against Jaguar Quitze, Jaguar Night, Not Right Now, and Dark Jaguar the nations were met with a walled fortification on top of which are what appear to be warriors. Having failed in stealing the three deities or managing to trick them, the nations have travelled up the mountain of the K'iche, and along the way the four mother-fathers prank them shaving the hair on their faces as they slept. The mother-fathers, meanwhile, have brought their wives and children to view the battle signaling their confidence in their power to overcome the nations, a confidence given to them by Tohil, Auilix, and Hacauitz. The nations surrounding the citadel soon realize that the warriors inside were simply manikins and they begin to bellow and howl, distorting their faces and whistling through their hands. The gourds of yellow jackets, wasps, and bees are released and the nations "were dazed by the yellow jackets and wasps. No longer able to hold on to their weapons and shields, they were doubled over and falling to the ground, stumbling. They fell down the mountain" (Tedlock 1996, 173). The nations meet defeat and are made "payers of tribute" having succumbed to the pain from the stings of the yellow jacket, wasp, and bee. Thwarted in their efforts to steal or trick the deities of the K'iche', and conquered rather than conquering them, the Nations succumbing to the pain of the stinging insects are brought low and they fail.

Pain, and its presence and absence, marks the failure of an act, venture, or event. Unlike kinship and speech, pain does not mark a boundary between human and non-human animals in the *Popol Vuh*, but instead functions as an indicator, a foreshadowing of a missing, a failure, of a being brought low and positioned as serving rather than being served. Such was the fate of non-human animals, the manikins, Seven Macaw, One and Seven Huanapu, and the nations. They suffered and were overcome by pain and as such signaled their failure and an essential lack that precludes the possibility of any success. Non-human animals suffer (and inflict) pain signifying their failure to fulfill the human design, a state brought about by their inability to speak the language of the deities, something the nations were equally incapable of doing. Only the four mother-fathers could converse with the deities Tohil, Auilix, and Hacauitz. The nations, like non-human animals, could not share speech with the deities. The nations succumb to pain and death when they are sacrificed to the deities, while non-human animals succumb to pain and death when they served as food. The presence of the indexical sign, pain, signifies those who fail, while its absence signifies those who succeed.

Boundaries and Borders

From the outset, the mythological texts examined, the Homeric epics and the *Popul Vuh*, the human and non-human animal are constituted as ontologically and metaphysically different; there is no possible kinship that links them with humans in creation. A second criterion, speech, is also central to marking the boundary between the human and non-human animal and marks those ontologically proper, the human animal, and those who are not, the non-human animal. The anthropogonic and demogonic myths examined above, like most ontological and sociogonic narratives, are foundational to the categories of the human and non-human animal and to the boundary located between them. This boundary is constructed by emphasizing what is already seen to be uniquely human, in the instance of this study, kinship speech, and pain. In this play, not surprisingly, the sign of the non-human animal signifies as lesser than the sign of the human animal, and like the boundary between, serves to secure the ontologically privileged place of the human animal. In the Maya *Popol Vuh*, however, if kinship and language demonstrated a ontological and metaphysical difference, pain plays a slightly different role, and although equally signifying as a negative, that is a signal of going wrong and/or failure, pain in this text speaks instead of a "being brought low," "serving," and a coming under the power of another in a hierarchical arrangement.

In terms of binarisms, both signs of human and animal only come to mean in relation to each other: the animal is what the human is not, the human is what the animal is not. Furthermore, in a binary play one sign is negatively valued, and the other is positively valued so the non-human animal signifies as negative and the human animal positive when in relation to each other. The binary relations are validated and given fundamental value in these mythological texts insofar as the texts act to provide reason and rationale for the relations between the non-human and human animal, relations of control, domination and subjugation deemed natural and normative in the *Iliad*, *Odyssey*, and *Popol Vuh*.

In light of the normativized and naturalized "knowledge" that non-human animals are subordinate to, serve, and are less than human animals, the human and non-human animal caesura is immeasurably useful for developing further demarcations within and without social bodies. Since anthropogonic and demogonic myths ground their narratives in the ontological and metaphysical, they are useful to forge boundaries between groups of people or kinds of people in the social body. And, since the ontological and metaphysical statuses of non-human and human animals in these kinds of myths are seen as essentially and irrevocably true, having been established in an authoritative mythological text, when analogically applied to those who would be made "other" internally (for example the Rohingya of Myanmar) or externally (for example, refugees) the play of social and political power is made invisible rooted as it is in so-called nature that is inserted via the animal/human binary. The boundary between non-human and human is securely rooted in a distant and unchanging mythic past and therefore beyond criticism. In the "proper order of things" (Foucault 1973), convention, the sign of the non-human animal and the boundary between it and the human animal have been and continue to be eminently useful for the ideological deployment of power.

In the Homeric myths, the lack of pain exhibited by classes of animals; that is those demarcated for sacrifice, labor, product, or food, allows for an absence of consideration of the pain of non-human animals and in this reinforces the boundary between animal and human. Succumbing to pain, seen in the texts, is an indication of failure, of a warrior who lacks proper masculinity or an act, event, or character destined to fail as in the *Popol Vuh*. Similarly, then, the presence of the indexical sign, pain, signifies a general lack: in the *Popol Vuh* the presence of pain itself signals or foreshadows failure and in this failure a lack on the behalf of those who have failed, such as the non-human animals who could not speak and count the days as required of them by the deities.

Chapter 3

Ancient Spartan Masculinities and Pain
A Case Study

> Memory speed to this lady
> our own muse, who knows
> about us and the Athenians,
> about the day at Artemisium
> when they spread sail like gods
> against the armada
> and defeated the Medes;
> while we were led by Leonidas,
> like a wild boar we were,
> yes, gnashing our tusks, our jaws running
> streams of foam, and our legs too.
> The enemy outnumbered the sands on the shore, those Persians.
> Goddess of the Wilds, Beast Killer,
> come this way maiden goddess,
> to join in the treaty,
> and keep us together for a long time.
>
> (Aristophanes, *Lysistrata* 1247–1265)

Introduction

In films such as *300*, released in 2007, and in the ancient world of Greece and later Rome, the mythography of the military and physical prowess of Spartan men, particularly their Spartan masculinity, figures as breathlessly awesome and a masculinity to be revered and imitated. Several ancient authors who act as primary sources for the Spartan "mirage," as Paul Cartledge (2001, 169–184) names it, are the Athenian Xenophon of the fifth to the fourth centuries BCE and Boeotian Plutarch of the first and second centuries CE, while those concerned with representations of Spartan masculinity more toward the dreadful are found in the writings attributed to Plato and Aristotle. Regardless of the variation of representation, they all agree that Spartan masculinity was acquired through a long, arduous and intermittently heavily ritualized engagement with pain; the indexical sign that incised the contours of masculinity onto the bodies of boys and youths as they became men within the Spartan disciplinary-educational system.

Pain appears to be intimately linked to the construction of masculinity in the context of Sparta. How is this achieved? Why pain? What is it about pain that it serves this function? To answer these questions I have developed a case study of the entwinement of pain and masculinity in ancient Sparta asking, what was/is the representation of proper Spartan masculinity? How was proper masculinity acquired/achieved? What was/is at stake in the proper performance of Spartan masculinity? What was/is the role of pain in the drama and performance of proper Spartan masculinity? Why pain? And particularly, why ritualized pain? To do this work I focus on narratives, both modern and ancient, wherein Sparta and Spartan masculinity are represented/imagined. I also draw on archeological texts that reference the tangible traces of Spartan ritual in the remains of altars and temples wherein the acquirement of proper masculinity was performed through the interplay of power and pain.

300, Pain, and Masculinity

The film *300*, released in 2007 and directed by Zack Snyder, presented an imaginative representation of an event that took place in 480 BCE wherein one of two kings of Sparta, Leonidas, took 300 of Sparta's best warriors (called *hippeis* or cavalry men although they were unhorsed) to face the Persians in a place called Thermopylea, or the "Hot Gates" as it translates into English (Cartledge 2007, ix). In the film we are presented with muscular and tough male Spartans, properly masculine; that is the beautiful warrior who seeks the beautiful death (Loraux 1977). The Spartan hoplites are presented as minimally clad wearing leather briefs, helmet, grieves, shield, cloak, and sandals, and carrying a sword. As the film was based on a comic book rendition of the story of this ancient event, it did not seek to be historically accurate, although it remained true to the event in general, and certainly captured the myth of Spartan warrior masculinity.

The opening narrative of the film introduces the viewer to infant Leonidas, the central figure in the film. The viewer is told, as a Spartan man with long gray hair stands on a precipice holding the infant Leonidas over a deep rocky crevice with a multitude of small bones and skulls, "When the boy was born ... like all Spartans, he was inspected. If he'd been small or puny or sickly or misshapen ... he would have been discarded." Shortly thereafter the viewer learns that at seven years of age Leonidas was inducted into the Spartan educational systems, the *agoge*; "taken from his mother and plunged into a world of violence ... Manufactured by 300 years of Spartan warrior society to create the finest soldiers the world has even known" (Snyder 2007). As the narrator relates this information the viewer is provided with images of young boys engaged in bloody fist fights, with the young Leonidas bleeding and beaten, but in the next shot we are presented with a bloody and unbeaten Leonidas: injured but victorious.

We next see an older Leonidas tied to a pillar and being beaten with a rod (suggestive of the *diamastigosis* of which I discuss later) as we learn that the boys and then youths are taught to show no response to pain. They must embrace pain and death in order that they not be subject to fear. Spartan male initiation, comments the narrator, meant being tossed into the wild to face whatever "nature" had to throw at the youth, with little other than one's own wits. In the film we are presented with the image of an adolescent with a long spear wearing little clothing climbing among the rocks as the wind and snow howl around him. Freezing, Leonidas is confronted by a monstrous wolf whom he slays and skins. Wearing the fur of his kill Leonidas returns to Sparta having more than successfully survived his "time in the wild" (this would appear to be a reference to the Krypteia). We then see him presented with a Spartan helmet and sword marking his Spartan masculinity; a warrior masculinity has been secured and is now recognized by his Spartan elders. Viewers are given to believe that it was precisely because of his proper Spartan warrior masculinity that Leonidas was able to stand against Xerxes and his massive Persian army. Leonidas was slain, along with his 300, because of the treachery of those men of Sparta who signified as neither warriors nor properly masculine.

The heroes of the film, Leonidas and his 300, are white, muscular, well-tressed, and are men of few words. Those men who are not properly masculine, and there are several in the film aside from Persians, speak too much, while their hair is shorn as imaged in the figure of the treacherous Counsellor Theron. It is Theron in the film who suggests diplomacy, that is using words instead of arms, and who is one of two traitors responsible for the defeat and death of Leonidas and his 300 warriors. The other improperly masculine figure is Ephialtes, whose misshapen body meant that his family had fled Sparta in order that he not be killed when an infant. Ephialtes is shown returning to Sparta and seeking to join Leonidas and his army of 300. Leonidas refuses him on pragmatic grounds, the outcome of which is Ephialtes's betrayal of the Spartans when he provides Xerxes with information about a path that leads behind the Spartan forces holding the pass. This deceit culminates in the death of Leonidas and his 300 Spartan warriors.

The figures of Theron and Ephialtes each represent failed masculinity and although not named as "tremblers" in the film, a Spartan concept applied to those deemed cowards, they represent this group of men who had failed to be fearless in battle, to protect the king and Sparta or to embrace the hard life of a properly masculine Spartiate. As Xenophon in the *Constitution of the Lacedaemonians* (10.7) wrote, "if someone, through cowardness, shrank from the hard effort required by the laws, he (Lycurgus) ordained that that man should no longer be reckoned a member of the *homoioi*"[1] (in Hodkinson and Powell 2006, 15). What is, beyond the physical markers of shorn hair and misshapen body, the signification of their lack? Their unwillingness to embrace pain: Theron visibly fears the Persian emissary and shrinks from him and his rod of kings' skulls, while Ephialtes refuses the painful truth of his inability to be a spartan warrior. Both refused pain and in so doing placed their feet on the path of a shameful death.

What was it that Leonidas and his 300 were willing to die for? In the film we are told it is freedom. From the first moment when the monstrous and effeminate Persian emissary asks King Leonidas to submit to Xerxes slavery and freedom are juxtaposed. The very orientalized Persians are presented as a social system made up of a vast "slave works," visually akin to Peter Jackson's rendition of J. R. R. Tolkien's Mordor, while the Spartans are represented as "truly" free men, unencumbered warriors whose proper masculinity allowed them to be truly free. In another moment in the film, Leonidas is shown troubled as the Ephors, represented in the film as old, corrupt and depraved priests, refuse to support his request to meet the Persian attack, giving Apollo's festival the Karneia as the reason. Worried, Leonidas does not sleep unsure what to do. Gorgo, his partner and queen, advises Leonidas saying, "It is not a question of what a Spartan citizen should do. Nor a husband, nor a king. Instead ask yourself, my dearest love ... what should a free man do" (Snyder 2007)?

Another instance of freedom acting as a central mytheme in the film is when Leonidas and his 300 are departing for Thermopylae or the "Hot Gates" to join other Greeks standing against the Persian invasion. Standing on the road surrounded by vast fields of ripen wheat, Leonidas addresses his friend and Captain, Artemis, asking if the 300 present have sons to carry on their name? As Artemis responds affirmatively, a young warrior, Astinos, the Captain's son, responds with "We are with you, sire! For Sparta, for freedom. To the death." Departing the fields of wheat, Gorgo calls her husband back, but not for a teary embrace; rather she exclaims, "Spartan! ... Come back with your shield or on it." The narrator then comments, "There's no room for softness, not in Sparta. No place for weakness. Only the hard and strong may call themselves Spartans. Only the hard, only the strong. We march. For our lands, for our families, for our freedoms. We march" (Snyder 2007). In all three instances, and there are certainly many other examples, freedom is given as the reason for this deployment of Spartan warriors—the few who will protect Sparta and the many Greeks who know freedom but are unwilling to "die" for it.

Gorgo, queen of Sparta and partner to Leonidas, is also presented as embodying Spartan ideals of strength and courage in the film. Although Gorgo, step-niece and wife of Leonidas, is not presented as a warrior herself, she too upholds and honors Spartan hoplite masculinity. When asked by the Persian emissary, how dare she speak to men about the business of men, she responds "Because only Spartan women give birth to real men" (Snyder 2007). It would appear Gorgo, meaning Gorgon,[2] is an appropriate queen and partner to Leonidas the lion.

Frank Miller's *300*

The film *300* was based on a five-issue comic book series of the same name, written by Frank Miller, with painted colors by Lynn Varley, published in 1998, and collected into a single volume the following year (Miller 2006). The work drew from ancient writers such as Herodotus (fifth century BCE) and Plutarch (first and second centuries CE). The graphic novel was released in a five-issue limited series comic in 1998 (Murray 2007, 12). Frank Miller also created the 1991 serialized comic *Sin City*, which was made into a film, *Frank Miller's Sin City*, in 2005. Miller has developed a number of serialized comics and consistent across his creative canvas is the exaggerated masculine: muscular, tough, unrelenting, brave, and most did not succumb to pain. The exaggerated masculine that moves through the worlds Miller creates is slave to no one or anything, while he embraces discomfort, pain, or death. Miller's masculine is the heroic masculine of the comic book genre, and like the masculine, the heroic feminine is equally idealized in his graphic novels. The heroic feminine can be either a beautiful victim in need of rescue or whose death requires revenge (for example Goldie in *Sin City*), or she is the phallic female, strong determined, ruthless, and equally an avenger of the oppressed and downtrodden. Electra, the name of which came from a heroine of ancient Greek myth, is one such figure found in Miller's work. These kinds of femininity ultimately augment the exaggerated masculine and provide rationale for the existence of the warrior. Gorgo is herself strong and able requiring a partner strong enough to properly dominate her since proper Spartiatae were dominated by no one, particularly women.

Both the film and the graphic novel create a story that in its formation of masculinity, specifically Spartan masculinity, erases the negative implications of the construction and maintenance of a warrior masculinity. The viewer/reader is presented with vivid images of thrashed, whipped, starved, bruised, and frozen bodies of boys and youths, but such pain is presented as the signs by which the boys will become properly masculine warriors. The presumed suffering of children—their torture and maiming—is absent from the page and the screen. Equally absent in both narratives is the slavery that Sparta built its warrior nation upon, the helots whose labor made possible the claim that only Spartan hoplites were warriors, trained to war and not to the field, the potter's wheel, or any other occupation that engaged Greeks of other poleis and other Spartan men.

Although Miller, also an executive producer of the film, does not name Xenophon or Plutarch as ancient sources for his graphic novel, the ancient Greek historian Herodotus (fifth century BCE) does appear to have been one of his ancient sources (Murray 2007, 12). The earlier 1962 film *The 300 Spartans*, directed by Rudolph Maté, also influenced Miller's work (Murray 2007, 12), while Maté had primarily drawn on Plutarch for his rendition of the Battle of Thermopylae (Nioloutsos 2013). Plutarch was heavily dependent on Xenophon for his narrative of Sparta allowing Xenophon also to make his way into the mythic construction of Spartan masculinity in Maté, then Miller, and finally Zack Snyder, the director of *300*. Spartan masculinity, by the time of the 2007 film, then, was already a complexly woven mythography. Although Herodotus provides some narrative on Sparta and its political and military doings, his Histories are more concerned with the doings of Greece in general than with Sparta in particular. Therefore, although in the following study Herodotus does comes up, particularly with regard to the battle of Thermopylae, my data for analysis of the myth of Spartan masculinity come primarily from Xenophon and Plutarch, both of whom are the principle ancient myth-makers of Spartan masculinity.

Plutarch and the Myth of Spartan Masculinity

The Greek historian and biographer Plutarch lived around 45–120 CE in Greece and he is a primary historical source for ancient Sparta. Plutarch wrote his biographies, *Parallel Lives*, where he developed studies of those he considered to be the great men of ancient Greece and Rome. In his biographies, Plutarch provides narrative on the lives, *bioi*, of four Spartan kings, Lycurgus, Agesilaus, Agis, and Cleomenes and while scholars believe Plutarch wrote a life of Leonidas, it has yet to be found (Cartledge 2007, 172). What scholars do have, however, are the sayings attributed to Leonidas in the "Apophthegmata Laconica" found in Plutarch's *Moralia* some of which was incorporated into the dialogue of Miller's graphic novel and Snyder's film.

Plutarch's view of the Spartans is similar to both Miller and Snyder when it comes to his representation of Spartan masculinity: that is the male citizen hoplite. Plutarch's "life" of Lycurgus (*c*.900–800 BCE), king of Sparta and legendary law-giver, provides a history of Sparta wherein there is a shift from chaos and anarchy to order because of the laws of Lycurgus. In Plutarch's narrative, Lycurgus travels from a disorganized Sparta, where his good efforts were slandered by political opponents, to Crete and then Asia comparing different forms of social organization and governance. In Crete he encountered an austere and simple way of life, and this way of life he compared to the Ionians of Asia, his next port of call, and found the latter to be excessive. As Plutarch wrote "just as a physician compares with healthy bodies [Cretan] those which are unsound and sickly [Asia]; he could then study the difference in their modes of life and forms of government" (Plutarch 2005, Lyc. 4.3). Even as Lycurgus saw excess among the Ionians, he was, according to Plutarch's text, introduced to Homer's poems while in Ionia, and these he brought back to Greece which were partnered with his new austere laws for Spartans. Plutarch then references Lycurgus's travels to Egypt, whereupon he saw the class of warriors, among other classes, and then to Libya, Iberia, and even as far as India. In the narrative, the hero, Lycurgus, imposed exile upon himself in order to secure peace in the always potentially chaotic Sparta. He travels further and further away from the center—Sparta—going south, west and then east, and from these places he secures the gifts (the law and wisdom) that brought the heroic Spartan warrior into existence.

Plutarch's text further relates that Lycurgus, having secured the gifts of the law and wisdom, returned to Sparta. Travelling home, seeing the illness of the Spartan body politic, Lycurgus journeyed to Delphi where he secured the support of Apollo in his plan to institute a law that would completely alter the Spartan social body. There was a concentrated reorganization of governance in Lycurgus's laws, such as the creation of the group called the Senate or Council Elders to allow for a balance between tyranny (kings) and democracy (populace). But along with political changes came the proposal to implement practices that would construct the proper Spartan masculine citizen, the Spartan hoplite warrior.

The Spartan hoplite warrior constructed in the period of Lycurgus, Plutarch wrote, came about by attacking luxury and wealth. To do this common messes were established, while gold and silver currency were rejected. This austerity, Plutarch's Lycurgus argued, was to be definitive of Spartan life as it would produce strong bodies and spirits in all those of Sparta but more so among the males who would become properly masculine through the Spartan education system. In Plutarch's texts it was the education system that was the primary site for the production of the noble masculinity of the Spartan hoplite warrior. According to Plutarch's mythography of Sparta, male children were taken at age seven from the family homes and grouped into companies where their every movement was under constant surveillance. Deprived of the comfort of clothing, shoes, and warm blankets the boys were taught endurance, and while exercising they were taught to obediently welcome pain. Furthermore, undernourished, the boys/youth had to find other avenues to secure food such as theft risking harsh punishment. Plutarch wrote that theft was encouraged, as it allowed for the development of stealth and ingenuity, but being caught brought great shame. Plutarch then related a story as an example of the Spartan masculinity that was inculcated in the young: a boy had concealed a stolen fox under his cloak, but rather than being caught he allowed the fox to disembowel him making no sound of pain (Lyc. 18.1). In the narratives of Spartan masculinity pain is central to the construction of proper masculinity, and succumbing to pain brought shame to the child but it was a shame that extended beyond the child and was shared by his cohort, mentor and family.

Plutarch wrote of three other Spartan kings in his *Parallel Lives*. Agesilaus (r. 400–360 BCE), Agis (r. 245–241 BCE), and Cleomenes (r. 235–223 BCE), the latter two of whom ruled during a time when Sparta and its warriors had been diminished, according to Plutarch, due to a falling away from an authentic masculine ethos of austerity, strength, endurance, and imperviousness to all pain. Instead Spartans had embraced a false feminine ethos that included greed, weakness, flabbiness, and terror of pain. Plutarch wrote that during the rule of Agis Spartan women controlled most of the wealth in Sparta (2000a, *Agis* 7.3), a common fear of Greek men in general, while rich, older Spartan men revelled in pomp and indolence and enriched themselves at the cost of fellow Spartans. Plutarch suggested that only seven hundred Spartiatae were left, and of these only one hundred owned land beyond their assigned lot of land (*Agis* 5.4). Agis, on the other hand, had, before his twentieth year, "set his face against pleasures ... observed sedulously the Spartan customs in his meals and baths and general ways of living, and declared that he did not want the royal power at all unless by means of it he could restore the ancient laws and discipline" (*Agis* 4). Agis's efforts, however, were not successful and he was strangled along with his mother Agesistrata and grandmother Archidamia, by the supporters of Leonidas II, who had returned to Sparta having been deposed by Agis's supporters.

Cleomenes was the son of Leonidas II, and although too young for marriage, he had been given Agiatis, widow of the now dead Agis, as his wife by his father. When Cleomenes came to kingship Sparta was under control of the Ephors, a group of five meant to oversee the rule of Sparta when the kings were in the field of war. Cleomenes was able to wrest power away from the Ephors and then set out, as Plutarch had him declare, "to rid Sparta of her imported curses, namely luxury and extravagance, and debts and usury, and those elder evils than these, namely poverty and wealth, he would have thought himself the most fortunate king in the world..." (Plutarch 2000b, *Cleom.* 10.4). Cleomenes, with his soldiers, committed suicide in Egypt as the beautiful death in the battlefield had been left behind when Cleomenes chose to flee to "fight another day," but that day never arrived. Plutarch's text relates that Ptolemy had given the order that Cleomenes's body should be hung up in a leather bag, while his children, mother, and all of the women of his house were to be put to death; a death they all faced, Plutarch wrote, with Laconic prowess (*Cleom.* 38–39).

Agesilaus, who ruled Sparta one hundred years earlier, had difficulty with the power of the *ephorate* and the *gerousia* or those male citizens (twenty-eight in total) over sixty years of age. Unlike his predecessors before, however, Plutarch related, Agesilaus sought their favor and included them in all his decisions (Plutarch 2004, *Ages.* 4.3-4). Agesilaus, unlike most Spartan kings (Leonidas was also an exception), was taken into the *agoge*, or the ritualized disciplinary education of the Spartan male children: he had not been in line to the throne having been both second born and lame. His fortunes, however, changed after the death of his brother and with the support of his mentor-lover Lysander, who had become enamored of Agesilaus "when he was among the so-called 'bands'" (*Ages.* 2.1). Agesilaus took the throne from the son of Agis and ruled for forty years.

Although Agesilaus was said to have had some problem with his legs, he could walk and indeed proved to be as tough and as properly masculine as any of the kings of Sparta. Plutarch's text makes a point of reassuring the reader concerning Agesilaus's masculinity by having others admire it. We read that he had been in the field of war for nearly two years and his enemies and friends were impressed by his austerity, moderation, and his willingness to suffer as his soldiers suffered. Agesilaus was indifferent to cold and heat "as if nature had given him alone the power to adapt himself to the seasons as God has tempered them" (*Ages.* 16.2). His herculean nature is mentioned again in Plutarch's text in reference to the battle between the Thebans and Spartans at Coronea. Here Agesilaus fought furiously so much so that although he was wounded multiple times he had to be dragged from the battlefield and wounded as he was, according to Plutarch, he refused his tent until he had himself assured that the Spartan dead had been returned from the battlefield (*Ages.* 19.1).

Agesilaus's rule included numerous wars and during his rule Sparta lost control of Messenia and came very close to being overrun by the Thebans. The loss of Messenia meant the loss of fertile lands and the enslaved helots who grew the crops, while Spartan territory was halved. According to Plutarch, Sparta's dominance in Greece came to an end, although certainly the fascination concerning Spartan masculinity did not as Plutarch attested with regard to the ritual of flagellation he witnessed at the altar of Artemis-Ortheia (*Lyc.* 18.1).

Xenophon's Foundational Myth of Sparta

A primary source for Plutarch's mythography of Sparta and Spartan masculinity was Xenophon (430–354 BCE), who lived almost five hundred years prior to Plutarch. Xenophon was an Athenian citizen of wealth and friend of Socrates, of whom he wrote. Xenophon left Athens in 401 BCE and joined other Greek soldiers commanded by the Persian governor Cyrus, who was defeated. During this failed expedition Xenophon met the Spartan King Agesilaus whom he joined and fought alongside at the battle of Coronea against the Athenians, his fellow citizens. For this he was banished but was given an estate by the Spartans, and although reconciled to Athens after the defeat of the Spartans in 371 BCE, he lived out the rest of his life in Corinth writing of Sparta and his great friend Agesilaus of whom he wrote "now concerning his high birth what greater and nobler could be said than this, that even today the line of his descent from Heracles is traced through the roll of his ancestors ... kings and sons of kings?" (Xenophon 1968a, *Ages.* 1.1)

Xenophon, like many Socratic thinkers, was enamored of Sparta's governance, the dual kingship, and the checks and balances of power between the three ruling groups of the kings, ephors and elders. Most particularly, however, he liked the way the Spartans constituted themselves as a people and citizens. Found primarily in *Constitution of the Lacedaemonians*, Xenophon, himself a military officer, lauds the laws of Lycurgus and the militarized social structure proposed therein, while the text of "Agesilaus" proposes Agesilaus as a living and breathing example of the law. According to Xenophon, Agesilaus is pious, beyond the reach of covetousness, neither glutton nor idle. Agesilaus embraced hard work and never chafed at "the summer's heat and the winter's cold," and even in passion showed self-control and moderation. His courage exceeded others, while his wisdom ruled his deeds and patriotism guided his efforts (*Ages.* 3–4). Gracious to all, he chose to live by the rules of Lycurgus and so died the beautiful death of a warrior. Wrote Xenophon:

> So complete was the record of his service to his fatherland that it did not end even when he died: he was still a bountiful benefactor of the state [payment for his military services to the Egypt was returned home with his body] when

he was brought home to be laid in his eternal resting-place, and, having raised up monuments of his virtue throughout the world, was buried with royal ceremony in his own land.

(*Ages.* 2.16)

In his text the *Constitution of the Lacedaemonians* Xenophon elaborates on the reason that the Spartans prospered as a people: adherence to the laws of Lycurgus. Xenophon's *Constitution* is less about political structure and more about social organization and an ethos of life. In line with this, then, Xenophon explains how young girls, like young boys, were in the Spartan context physically trained to be strong. Nor should they be taught, wrote Xenophon, idle crafts such as carding wool since Lycurgus considered such activities sedentary and not proper for freeborn women whose primary role was to reproduce the next generation of Spartiatae (Xenophon 1968b, *Const. Lac.* 1.4).

Likewise found in Xenophon's narrative of Sparta (not surprising since Xenophon was a primary source for Plutarch) is a description of the Spartan education system, the *agoge*. This system, the text emphasizes, is one of the means by which Spartan boys become Spartan warriors:

> Instead of each father to appoint a slave to act as tutor, [Lycurgus] gave the duty of controlling the boys to a member of the class from which the highest offices are filled, in fact to the "Warden" as he is called. He gave this person authority to gather the boys together, to take charge of them and to punish them severely in case of misconduct. He also assigned to him a staff of youths provided with whips to chastise them when necessary; and the result is that modesty and obedience are inseparable companions at Sparta.
>
> (*Const. Lac.* 2.2)

Although the term *agoge* is typically translated as education, Jean Ducat makes a convincing argument that "discipline" is equally implied in the term and therefore translation of *agoge* as both education and discipline describes better the Spartan institution (2006a, 69); an institution for the making of the properly masculine Spartiatae. In the *agoge* boys were hardened via multiple mechanisms of pain as proposed in the laws Lycurgus. Unshod, one garment, food enough not to starve, the boys must learn to live with pain as a daily companion. Should, however, the boys find and take food, as warriors find and take the spoils of war, they had succeeded in part of their education. But should they be caught, they were soundly punished as stealth, cunning, and courage were required for successful theft and those who failed at it also failed at their education (*Const. Lac.* 2.3–9).

When the boys became youth, they next faced ceaseless labor, labor for Sparta and its occupants. When not working they were to be reticent, eyes downcast and modest in every respect (*Const. Lac.* 3.1-4). As they grew older the young men were organized into groups, while groups were set in agonistic relationship with each other. Three of the "best" young men were chosen by the ephors to be commanders, each with a rule of 100 men they subsequently chose. According to Xenophon, those not chosen were evermore at war with those who had secured these honors (*Const. Lac.* 4.3-4).

Securing adulthood, Spartiatae were to concern themselves with the business of freemen, which was, according to Lycurgus, labor that maintained civic freedom (*Const. Lac.* 8.1-3). The Spartiate was to be a citizen-soldier, one who chose "an honourable death in preference to a disgraceful life" (*Const. Lac.* 9.1). Provided with a "red cloak" since it least resembled women's clothing, and a bronze shield, the younger Spartiatae were allowed to wear their hair long so that when they made ready for battle they might comb their long locks, wreath their heads, and polish their shields to the music of the flutes (*Const. Lac.* 11.3). Theirs was to be a joyous march to victory and/or death. For Xenophon, then, the rule of Lycurgus defined the system of discipline and education that was the site of the construction of Spartan warrior masculinity.

Those male Spartans who failed the tests of masculinities enacted in the disciplinary-education system, a system that was highly ritualized, were defined as a group unto themselves. Xenophon wrote:

> But in Lacedaemon everyone would be ashamed to have a coward with him at the mess or to be matched with him in a wrestling bout. Often when sides are picked for a game of ball he is the odd man left out: in the chorus he is banished to the ignominious place; in the streets he is bound to make way; when he occupies a seat he must needs give it up, even to a junior; he must support his spinster relatives at home and must explain to them why they are old maids: he must make the best of a fireside without a wife, and yet pay forfeit for that: he may not stroll about with a cheerful countenance, nor behave as though he were a man of unsullied fame, or else he must submit to be beaten by his betters. Small wonder, I think, that where such a load of dishonour is laid on the coward, death seems preferable to a life so dishonoured, so ignominious.
>
> (*Const. Lac.* 9.4-6)

The "trembler" marked failed Spartan masculinity and so acted as a means by which to determine successful Spartan masculinity. The "trembler" as a figure of disgrace appears in the poetry of Tyrtaeus, a Laconian poet of the eighth century BCE. As a legal term that incurred state punishment, Jean

Ducat argues, *tresantes* or tremblers did not appear until Diodorus in the first century BCE and subsequently in the writings attributed to Plutarch (Ducat 2006b, 10). These later texts represent the enactment of state punishment wherein those found guilty of running away from battle were excluded from holding offices, from marriage contacts, and had to visibly mark themselves as tremblers requiring that one-half of the face be shaved and the other side unshaven. Their clothing was also to be unkempt and dirty (*Ages.* 30.3–4). Although the term may not have had a legal function, it had a social function so that public censure accompanied fleeing a battle or post, leaving the king unguarded, and throwing down one's arms. The fifth-century BCE historian Herodotus commented on this social censure when he wrote how Aristodemos, who left Leonidas at the battle of Thermopylae due to illness, faced social censure until he redeemed himself in the battle of Platea: "no Spartan would kindle fire for him, no one addressed a word to him, and he had the mortification of being called Aristodemos the Trembler" (in Ducat 2006b, 3). The trembler was everything the Spartiate was not, and as denigrated as the trembler was the successful warrior was elevated. The heroic warrior was lauded in the streets and participated in the ritual celebrations of the collective. The trembler was excluded from those practices that marked Spartiatae as equals among each other, while the trembler (his family also suffered his fate) held an inverted status of the enslaved helot:

> And he laid on the people the duty of practising the whole virtue of a citizen as a necessity irresistible. For to all who satisfied the requirements of his code he gave equal rights of citizenship, without regard to bodily infirmity or want of money. But the coward who shrank from the task of observing the rules of his code he caused to be no more reckoned among the peers.
>
> (*Const. Lac.* 10.7)

Plutarch's narrative of ancient Sparta and its manly men is a mythography wherein the great law-maker Lycurgus brought the Spartans from a state of chaos to one of order. This order he linked directly to a heroic masculinity instilled in its people, but most particularly in the boys, youths, and men who are made into warriors in the *agoge*. This kind of training is coupled with the rejection of comfort, luxury and wealth, the Spartan austerity, which is central to the kind of masculinity the texts attributed to Plutarch represent as Spartan. The rejection of wealth and its attendant weaknesses of lust, softness, and servility Plutarch ascribed to Lycurgus and his efforts to establish a powerful and just system of governance in Sparta. Obedience to the law of Lycurgus ensured, Plutarch argued, the continued power and dominance of

Sparta. As he wrote in *Agis*: "[n]ow, at this time the greater part of the wealth of Sparta was in the hands of the women, and this made the work of Agis a grievous and difficult one" (7.3). Two things found in Sparta were problematic and indicative of its decline, wealth (5.3) and rule by women. The Sparta of Lycurgus and its god-like warriors had been lost to the depths of time.

Xenophon's mythography of Sparta and the masculinity of its Spartiatae moved around the ideas of courage, wisdom, moderation, patriotism, discipline, modesty and bravery, all of which he wrote were secured by a willingness to endure pain rather than face the shame that accompanied those Spartans who turned their backs on battle. Xenophon wrote that "Thus his regulations with regard to the begetting of children were in sharp contrast with those of other states. Whether he succeeded in populating Sparta with a race of men remarkable for their size and strength anyone who chooses may judge for himself" (Const. Lac. 1.10). Those who lacked the courage to be Spartiatae, wrote Xenophon, occupied the position of "trembler" one he described as being shunned in Sparta, and who must give way to even junior men, whose wife has left his fire, who daughters remain unmarried, and who "must submit to being beaten by his betters" (*Const. Lac.* 9.4–5). Xenophon suggested that it is "[sm]all wonder ... that where such a load of dishonour is laid on the coward, death seems preferable to a life so dishonoured, so ignominious" (*Const. Lac.* 9.6). The process of making the Spartiate was one wherein boys were taught not to succumb to fear of pain or death, but instead to embrace them:

> He made it a point of honour to steal as many cheeses as possible [from the altar of Artemis-Ortheia], but appointed others to scourge the thieves, meaning to show thereby that by enduring pain for a short time one may win lasting fame and felicity. It is shown herein that where there is need of swiftness, the slothful, as usual, gets little profit and many troubles.
>
> (*Const. Lac.* 2.9)

It was for these reasons that Xenophon turned both his sons over to the Spartan *agoge* system.

Pain and Ritual Practices

Apollo and Artemis are two deities linked to youth in Sparta as well to youth in general throughout ancient Greece. In Sparta three festivals related to Apollo, the Hyakinthia, the Gymnopaidiai, and the Karneia, involved Spartan children and youth. Michael Petterssen (1992) argues that the three festivals together acted to mark the passage of young male Spartans as they moved through the highly ritualized disciplinary education system. Paul Cartledge argues the Spartan education system shared aspects with educational systems throughout Greece, that is male (and female in Sparta) children were taught reading, writing, music, dance and physical exercise. However, in Sparta education was compulsory for all children of the Spartiatae, even those fathered on helot mothers, to enter the *agoge* (Xenophon 1918, V. 3.10). The only male children exempt were those in line to take up kingship. Although there is a lack of certainty as to age classes as they moved through the Spartan *agoge*, most scholars agree that male children were taken into the system around the age of seven years. They remained within the *agoge* until the age of eighteen years whereupon they became liminal-like figures who served Sparta on its periphery guarding its borders, hunting with stealth and remaining unseen. Surviving this last test of endurance, at twenty years of age they joined their assigned mess (Cartledge 2001, 85).

Throughout their schooling violence and pain were the primary pedagogical tools by which to shape "soft" Spartan boys into "hard" Spartan warriors. Refusing children foot gear, for example, was understood to toughen their feet allowing them to be able to endure the harsh conditions one faced as citizen-warrior protecting Sparta. Ritualized bare-handed fist-fighting, flagellation, ball, chorus, and dance *agōnes*, possibly naked under the heat of the sun, tested and conditioned the boys, youths, and young men as part of their training to take up the role of the Spartiate whose craft was war.

The festival of the Hyakinthia was thought to have lasted three days and was one of the more important festivals in Sparta (Ducat 2006a, 262; Pettersson 1992, 10). It more than likely took place in the month of Hyakinthios (thought to be a summer month) as months tended to take the name of the most important festival or cult practice of the month (Pettersson 1992, 10 n.9). The deity associated with the festival was Apollo, while the hero was Hyakinthos, the beloved young man whom Apollo inadvertently killed with a throw of the discus. The possibly three-day festival, called the Amyklaion, was celebrated at the sanctuary of Apollo at Amyklai about five kilometers from Sparta (ibid., 10). The festival included all age groups in Sparta and began in an atmosphere of dread that included a sacrifice to the chthonic Hyakinthos. Midway through the festival the dread evaporated and was replaced by exuberance with choral singing, the dancing of archaic dances, and flute and kithara playing. Girls rode in chariots and boys on horses, while both groups participated in horse-races (ibid.; Ducat 2006a, 263). Michael Pettersson argues that the Hyakinthia was the first of three festivals and served as a rite of separation and shifting the boys/youth into a liminal state wherein they began their long journey to adulthood. The boys, at this time, enter the *agoge* and were then subject to the hierarchy of males wherein their actions came under praise or censure, both accompanied in one way or another by pain.

The second festival, the Gymnopaidiai served to mark further rites of passage argued Pettersson. It was a favourite festival in Greece and drew many visitors to Sparta. It is thought to have been held in August and more than likely consisted of choir and dance competitions between age classes of males; *paides* (seven–nineteen), *hebontes* (twenty and twenty-nine) (Ducat 2006a, 272), *andres* (thirty plus), and *gerontes* (sixty plus) (Pettersson 1992, 50) performed on part of the agora known as the *choros* or "the dancing ground" (Ducat 2006a, 267; Pettersson 1992, 43). The agonistic event also included a ball-game and boxing matches, both of which were sites for the delivery and reception of pain. Honouring Apollo Pytheaus (Ducat 2006a, 266), the male singers and dancers of the Gymnopaidiai performed without clothing (ibid., 272-273; Pettersson 1992, 47) and under the heat of the summer sun leading ancient sources and many scholars to suggest that the performances linked to this festival were trials of endurance (Pettersson 1992, 46-47; Cartledge 2001, 87), a frequent theme found in the ancient sources who describe the world of ancient Sparta. The ball game, or the *Spairomachia*, said to take place during the Gynnopaidiai, was named an *agon* and appears to be competitive play among older youth who, according to Pausanias, had ceased being *ephebes* and began to be counted among men (in Pettersson 1992, 46). Pettersson indicates the game appears to have consisted of the use of sticks and a ball, and while the game is unclear, players were said to strike each other (ibid., 46-47). Boxing matches were also a part of the festival; the capacity to endure the marking of the body with the indexical sign, pain, seemed to have been the underlying theme of the festival.

The Karneai is the most obviously military of the three coming of age festivals. The festival was celebrated in other Doric centers and although the timing of the Karneai is uncertain, Petterssen argues that the month of *Karneios*, the festival's namesake, fell in the late summer—August/September—and may well have represented the new year in Sparta linked as it was to the fall equinox (1992, 57-58 n.323).The festival is said to have lasted nine days (Ducat 2006a, 274) and appears to have been overseen and enacted by marriageable males (ibid., 275; Pettersson 1992, 57). At the center of the festival was Apollo Karneios or Apollo the ram, an image found on coins dated to 425-390 BCE (Pettersson 1992, 61-62; Graf 2009, 117). What all the events of the festival were is unclear, but what has been suggested by ancient authors is that there was: a sacrifice of the ram and its consumption; dance and musical competitions; a theatrical military base camp; and a foot pursuit or race (Graf 2009, 117-120; Pettersson 1992, 57-58).

Two significant features of the Karneai commented on by ancient authors were the theatrical military encampment and the foot pursuit/race. Pettersson takes the theatrical theatre of arms at rest to be an imitation of military training and what the theatre represented above all was obedience with every action in the festival "done on command of a herald" (Demetrios of Skepsis in Pettersson 1992, 57). The pursuit, however, seems unconnected to the military ritual and scholars have argued that this aspect could well represent an earlier layer of Spartan history wherein the harvest was emphasized, particularly the grape harvest. Others saw the pursuit/race as an expiatory rite, a ritual drama, wherein the guilt of warfare was assuaged (Pettersson 1992, 60).

Pettersson argues for a different understanding of the pursuit/race. The ritual performance of the pursuit consisted of a man wearing woolen fillets proclaiming blessings on the city as he was pursued by young men called *staphylodromoi* or grape runners (Graf 2009, 119). Catching him meant good fortune for Sparta, while not catching him meant ill fortune. Pettersson understands the rite to be linked to divination and the seer, particularly in light of how important knowing the will of the deities was to ancient Greeks. The seer, of course, was linked to Apollo. Pettersson notes that seers held a place of privilege among the Spartans and a seer was attached to the king's staff. The kings, such as Leonidas, led the army and with them went those who could read the sacrifices, of which three took place when the army was on the move; "before departure, at the borders of the country and before the battle" (Pettersson 1992, 69). Having the seer among one's weaponry when going to war was necessary and indeed central to success.

Often connected to these three Apollonian festivals are two other Spartan rites considered important to the construction of Spartan masculinity, and clearly linked masculinity to pain, suffering, and endurance: the theft of cheese and scourging were combined at the altar of Artemis-Ortheia; and the Krypteia, a rite that consisted of young men soon to be hoplite warriors who occupied interstitial space hiding during the day, living off the land and supposedly hunting helots or the Messenians whom the Spartans had enslaved to grow their crops and provide their everyday needs since warriors had no time for such labors. The Krypteia has had various descriptions by ancient authors. Plutarch rejects Lycurgus as the founder of the Krypteia and instead argues that it was a later rite that came into practice possibly after the earthquake and subsequent revolt of the Messenians in the fifth century BCE (Lyc. 28.5). Plutarch judged the practice to be nefarious and primarily focused on the murdering of helots. The hunt appears to have been a rite wherein Spartan magistrates selected a group of young warriors whom they armed each with a dagger and sent into the wild places to watch the road in order to ambush and kill helots they might see on it. Plutarch also wrote that these warriors attacked and killed any helots considered to be a threat to Spartan domination.

Plato, Aristotle, and a scholion on Plato's *Laws* 1.633b–c comprise the other ancient sources that reference the Krypteia. Plato represents the Krypteia as "severe training in hardihood, as the men go bare-foot in winter and sleep without coverlets and have no attendants, but wait on themselves and rove through the whole countryside both by night and by day" (Plato 1967, 1.633b–c). Aristotle, on the other hand, is credited with saying that the warriors of the Krypteia "even to this day ... go out of the city to hide by day, and by night in arms ... and slaughter helots as they think necessary" (in Ducat 2006a, 284). The ninth century CE scholion to Plato (ibid., 289) while repeating what is written in the *Laws*, adds further information and informed the reader that in the Krypteia a young man was sent out to survive in the wild by his wits. The scholiast wrote that the initiate endured this harsh life for a year and for the entire duration the initiate must remain undetected as detection brought punished (Ducat 2006a, 289; see also Cartledge 2001, 88).

The *diamastigosis,* or ritual flogging held at the altar of Artemis-Ortheia, appears to be a later form of an earlier Spartan rite wherein male youth—Petterssen argues fourteen to seventeen years of age (1992, 85)—must steal cheeses from the altar of Artemis while dodging lashes. Those who secured the most cheese won the *agon*. By the time of Plutarch, however, the rite consisted of youths moving around the altar of Artemis and presenting their backs to be lashed again and again as long as they could endure the pain. Those who endured the most pain won (Ducat 2006a, 249–251), while the stealing of cheese was no longer a part of the rite. For Xenophon, the rite was a means by which to teach young men not to fear pain, but to embrace it in order to achieve the desired ends (*Const. Lac.* 2.2). This rite appears to have been connected to the beginning of military training in the *agoge*, the training of which began where they were about fourteen years of age (Pettersson 1992, 85).

Archeological Remains: The Sanctuary of Artemis-Ortheia

The sanctuary of Artemis-Ortheia (the meaning of Ortheia is "upright" or "erect" and is connected to the *xoanon*, a large wooden carving, of Ortheia) was located in the Spartan demos of Limnes south of Sparta proper. Artemis had at least thirty-one active sanctuaries in Laconia and nine in Sparta proper (Brulotte 2002, 180). The sanctuary of Ortheia is dated to at least the ninth century BCE (Cartledge 2001, 172–173; Ducat 2006a, 196), with pottery and remains dating to the tenth century BCE, and was dedicated to Ortheia, with earlier forms of the name being *Wortheia* and *Worthasia*. Ortheia's clear connection to Artemis does not appear until the first century CE (Carter 1987, 375). It appears that it was in circa 700 BCE that Sparta, having enslaved the Messenians, reformed its constitution, introduced the ephorate, which acted as a check to the power of the Spartan kings, and rebuilt, for the first time, the sanctuary of Artemis-Ortheia.

Archeologists have noted a number of reconstruction projects at this sanctuary over the hundreds of years it was used apparently due to flooding or destruction. It was during the Roman period that a quasi-amphitheater was built in association with the sanctuary (Cartledge 2001, 172). According to Paul Cartledge, scholar of all thing Laconic, "at the height of Sparta's power in the 6th to the 4th centuries BCE," the sanctuary of Ortheia contained a Doric temple, a stone-faced altar, and a number of buildings thought to store ritual paraphernalia and accoutrements, offerings, and so forth (Cartledge 2001, 172–173).

Found in the earliest levels of the sanctuary are pottery shards and animal bones (900 BCE), while ivory and bronze figurines, lead votive offerings, terracotta masks, and stelai, referencing victors of the *paidikoi agōnes* who dedicate the sickle they had won to Ortheia (Pettersson 1992, 82), turn up in later deposits beginning in the late seventh century BCE (Cartledge 2001, 177). The sickle, the earliest dedication dated to the classical period (Ducat 2006a, 210–212), appears to have been the "weapon" the boys were given once they began the *agoge* (ibid., 210; Pettersson 1992).

The terracotta masks are also curious and although some suggest they may have been worn by the boys in procession to or from Ortheia's altar (Ducat 2006a, 255) or in association with the ritual activity at the altar (Carter 1987, 356),[3] others have argued the masks would have been too heavy, visually limiting, even with cut-out eyes, and cumbersome to be worn as a mask in procession or in ritualized dance, choir or theatre performance. Instead, Jonah Rosenberg argues that the terracotta masks buried at the sanctuary of Artemis-Ortheia were copies of functional masks of malleable material, painted and used in ritual dramatic performance, possibly farce and mime, at the altar of Ortheia, but he does not link the masks with the boys in procession (2015, 257–259).[4]

The masks come in a number of different types with scholars suggesting seven to four or even two types (Carter 1987, 356). Jane Carter discusses types of masks in her article "The masks of Ortheia"; "furrowed grotesques, heroes, satyrs and gorgons," although satyrs and gorgons she subsequently locates under "furrowed grotesques" arguing masks of satyrs and gorgons, like the furrowed grotesque masks, also play on the monstrous (ibid., 358). Because there are holes along the edge of the "masks" scholars have taken this to mean the masks were possibly worn. However, the perforations could also have been for the addition of head and facial hair to the masks. The hero's mask is smooth of face and although seemingly blank in expression, the blankness is meant to suggest, Carter argues, ease of heart and mind. The hero mask signifies a state of being unperturbed and tranquil. The furrowed grotesque masks, on the other hand, have etched lines of pain and grief around their mouths, on their foreheads and across their cheeks. Although age may be one of the significations for the furrows, another viable reading is pain and suffering. The masks' furrows are deep and disfigure the faces and even as the hero mask is unmarked by the passage of pain, the furrowed grotesque masks are drenched with it.

The sickle is another artifact found at Artemis-Ortheia's sanctuary. Pettersson (1992, 83) argues that the sickle, called a *drepanon* by some, was an ancient military weapon. Pettersson notes that Jean-Pierre Vernant (1991, 234 n. 29) argued the implement has been mistakenly taken to be an agricultural tool and is instead a weapon, a short curved blade, used by the young as well as used during the Krypteia (Pettersson 1992, 84, 89). Jean Ducat (2006a, 213–214) comments in his text that the sickle is both a weapon and an agricultural tool and both uses are fit for non-warriors such as male children in the process of becoming warriors. Ducat also notes, drawing on Uta Kron's work, that the sickle in Greek myth came into play when a young—*ephebe*—male hero was faced with a monstrous opponent they must overcome. Kronus's emasculation of Ouranos and Perseus's slaying of Medusa were both done with a sickle, and instantiate this motif (ibid., 214).

Uta Kron's article "Sickles in Greek Sanctuaries: Votives and cultic instruments" notes that sickles have been in evidence since the early neolithic with the emergence of cereal-growing agriculture. Bronze and iron sickles are found among the Minoans and Mycenaeans, and iron sickles are found in ancient Greece well down into the Roman period (Kron 1998, 188–189). The sickles that were figured on stelai or the few remaining metal examples found at the sanctuary of Ortheia were slightly curved, often equipped with a handle and sometimes have a dent in the center of its blade (ibid., 194). Called "*harpe, drepane, drepanon,* and perhaps *aichme*," the sickle turns up in graves, sanctuaries, and less frequently in settlement sites (ibid., 195).

At the altar of Ortheia were found stelai recording the names of male youths who had won the competitions held in association with the Ortheia altar and had been awarded an iron sickle, which they dedicated to Ortheia. Kron writes that the sickles were connected to a series of competitions that comprised the *paidikoi agōnes* and consisted of three competitions; the *moa*, *kelea*, and *kassertorion*. Based on the meaning of the names, the first two are thought to possibly have been musical competitions and the last is considered to have been a hunting game (Kron 1998, 201). Petterssen argues that the age class of fourteen through to seventeen participate in these competitions at the altar of Ortheia (1992, 85).

The sickle is central to a number of mythical narratives aside from those of Ouranos and Medusa, both decapitated with this archaic weapon. The great Heracles, ancestor to the Spartans, with his younger nephew, Iolaos manages to kill the many-headed hydra with the sickle, the weapon carried by the ephebe Iolaos (Kron 1998, 190–191). Hermes, as an ephebe, also used to sickle in order to kill Argos, the monster appointed by Hera to stand between Io and Zeus (ibid., 193). Consistent in these myths is the use of a sickle as a weapon by a young, beardless male hero who has yet to achieve adulthood, but who may well achieve it by succeeding in the test at hand.

The altar of Ortheia and its accompanying masks and sickles, and its clear references to gendered rites of passages acted, and continues to act, as an anchor for the mythologies of Spartan warrior and trembler masculinities. The site and activities associated with it are spoken of by both Xenophon and Plutarch, as well as by Plato (*Laws* 1.633b), and are linked to ritual games called the *paidiakoi agōnes*. There is reference to the ritual of cheese theft from the altar where male youth must secure cheeses and endure lashings to do so, and the possibly later (Ducat 2006a, 251) ritual flagellation on the altar that Plutarch comments on in his works. Aside from boys' rites of passage, the altar was also the site of girls' rites of passage, probably similar to the boys in terms of choral and dance competitions. Alcman, the seventh to the sixth century Spartan poet known for the *partheneia*, wrote for the Spartan girl choirs, and the writings attributed to him make reference to the robe, called a plough, made by the girls and brought by them to the altar of Ortheia (Kron 1998, 203). Upon reaching the altar they appear to have sang of their beauty and desirability (Campbell 1982–1993, 365, 367).

Analysis

The data I have drawn on to speak of the myth of Spartan warrior masculinities, and pain as the indexical sign central to it, begin in the twentieth and twenty-first centuries with the film and graphic novel. These constructions of the myth of Spartan masculinity drew on Plutarch of the first and second centuries CE whose construction of Spartan masculinity drew on the work of Xenophon, the Athenian noble of the fifth and fourth centuries

BCE. Also linked to the mythical constructions are the Spartan festivals and rites that appear to have drawn much attention from other Greeks: the Hyakinthia, Gymnopaidiai, Karneia, the often reference Krypteia and the altar of Artemis-Ortheia, the ritual use of which has been dated to circa 700 BCE, while the site served as a sanctuary beginning in the tenth century BCE (Boardman 1963, 2).

Zack Snyder's film presents a visual/textual narrative of Spartan masculinity: the visual of muscular men clad in little other than leather briefs and red cloaks. Their hardened bodies do not respond to the environment around them as they were, through the endurance of pain, able to transcend what others could not. Marked as hypermasculine, particularly against the orientalized Persians whose feminine affectations, represented by their excessive and ornamental dress evidenced in the group of the masked and cloaked Immortals and the jewel-encrusted body of Xerxes, Spartan masculinity, signified as proper masculinity in Snyder's film, eschewed excess, opulence, and concealment and instead stand exposed to all, including the elements in their "nakedness." Spartan warrior masculinity is as simple and transparent as the Spartan warriors are unclothed. In the film and novel this is the natural and normative state for men who are true to their masculine natures.

Snyder's Spartan masculinity also includes several other attributes that add to the mythology not found in Plutarch or Xenophon; the insistence of heteronormativity, and the rejection of religion and ritual and instead an embracing of reason and rationality linked to law and freedom. The rejection of religion, that is the rejection of the ephors who are presented in the film as lustful and deceitful priests who betrayed Sparta and Leonidas to Xerxes, is also found in Miller's graphic novel and appears to be something both mythographers were very interested in representing. Represented as necessary to achieve freedom was the choice of rationality over and against "religion" represented as enslavement.

Freedom, as represented in film and novel, was a state of being achieved by Proper Spartan warriors who are represented as subject to none and living free, but to live free they must be willing to obey Spartan law and embrace "a beautiful death": "And by Spartan law, we will stand and fight ... and die. A new age has begun. An age of freedom. And all will know that 300 Spartans ... gave their last breath to defend it" (Snyder 2007).

From the perspective of the twentieth and twenty-first centuries it was the Spartans who fought for freedom for themselves and all Greeks, and subsequently modern humanity's freedom from the corrupting "east" as represented by Xerxes and his Persian army. In Snyder and Miller's representations of Spartan masculinity, freedom is definitive of the truly masculine male, and the Spartan males in film and graphic novel are unencumbered by work, women, children, and even bodily needs. Instead they stand every ready for battle, or rather those who were properly masculine. Older men in the film, possibly the gerousia, which was made up of Spartiatae sixty years and older who had finished their military service and provided direction to the kings, are shown accompanying Theron; the central traitor in the film who is depicted as in collusion with Persians against Sparta, or at least against Leonidas and Gorgo, the queen of Sparta. These older men are presented as fearful, easily swayed, and like the ephorate, compromised by their lack of masculinity in that they are slaves to fear and death, and therefore neither free nor Spartiatae.

Men who are not properly masculine, and therefore not Spartiatae, are weak and therefore easily corruptible. The ephorate are depicted as ruled by their lust and greed. They too have been bought by the Persians, and so they insist that the festival of the Karneia must go forward, which meant that Sparta could not go to war against the Persians. Leonidas, properly cynical, rejects the ruling of the ephors and departs with his personal guard of 300, to hold back the Persians (Snyder 2007; Miller 2006). Leonidas's cynicism is not simply expressed by him, but equally by the narrator, Dilios, who commented that, when Leonidas sought to convince the ephorate that Sparta must go to war against Xerxes and the Persians, "[t]here's never been a *holy man who lacked the love of gold*" and again that they were "*remnants of the old times ... before Lykurgos the law-giver ... Before Sparta's ascent from the age of Darkness*" (Miller 2006, emphasis original). Properly masculine Spartiatae do not believe in gods or ancient ritual, but they do obey the law and so obey these "moldy, rotting *remnants* of ancient, senseless *stupid* tradition" (ibid., emphasis original).

Should the viewer of the film think that the properly masculine Spartiatae such as Leonidas were the atheists of the ancient world, they would be quite mistaken. Leonidas did march with only 300, according to ancient mythographers, but not because religion and reason came into conflict; rather upon the completion of the Karneia the entirety of the army was to be sent. The Karneia honored Apollo Karneios (as ram) and, as Petterssen notes, celebrated militarism and military life along with a race by young men to capture the "*staphylodromoi,*" the man wrapped in fillets of wool who ran through the city crying out good omens. The capture of the "*staphylodromoi*" brought the city good luck (Petterssen 1992, 68). Sparta was known for its adherence to ritual and indeed did not march without a seer and would perform sacrifices during the entire expedition. Both Plutarch and Xenophon comment on the piety of the Spartans and consider it a mark of their superiority as a people.

Xenophon wrote that when the Spartiatae saw the enemy, they would make a sacrifice and "custom ordains that all the flute players present are to play and every Lacedaemonian is to wear a wreath. An order is also given to polish arms. It is the privilege of the young warrior to comb his hair before entering battle, to look cheerful and earn a good report" (*Const. Lac.* 13.8–9). Ritual and deities like Zeus, Apollo, the Dioscuri, and Athena were important to securing success in the field of war, while Artemis ensured the success in raising the young (Budin 2016).

Equally central to Miller's and subsequently Snyder's representation of Spartiatae, and therefore Spartan masculinity, is pain. The indexical sign pain establishes a link between the material of ritual and the symbolic of language. C. S. Peirce has convincingly argued that "an index is a sign which would, at once, lose the character which makes it a sign if its object were removed, but would not lose that character if there were no interpretant" (1991, 239). That is, the mark of its passage would remain. Equally so with the indexical sign of pain: if the fist, the whip, the cold, or the sickle were removed pain would lose its character; but pain would not lose its character if the interpretant was absent. The indexical sign-function does not impute a direct connection to the object even if described as contiguous with its object, that is, "'whose relation to their objects consists in a correspondence of fact'" (Peirce in Sebeok 1994, 65). The relationship, rather, is rhetorical and employs metonymy to provide a sense of contiguity. Indexical signs also have "'the being of present experience'" (Peirce in Sebeok 1994, 63), and "furnish positive assurance of the nearness and reality of their Objects. But with the assurance there goes no insight into the nature of those Objects" (Peirce 1991, 251–252).

In terms of its object, the indexical sign does not share characteristics with it, nor is it similar. Rather, Peirce explains:

> [I]t is in dynamical (including spatial) connection with the individual object, on one hand, and with the senses or memory of the person whom it serves as a sign, on the other hand. Let it be recalled that all objects, on the one hand, and the memory being the reservoir of interpretants, on the other hand, are also kinds of signs or systems of signs.
>
> (Peirce in Sebeok 1994, 65)

Equally, with the indexical sign there is a secondness whereby that which is there intrudes and pushes in appearing as "an external fact of another something" (Peirce 1991, 185).

In Miller's graphic novel the first pages present an army on the move, and the first action within the moving body of men in red cloaks is the failure of a young hoplite, who after three days marching in extreme heat stumbles and falls only to bring about derision and punishment from the Captain who began to beat the young man, the latter who willingly accepted his punishment. The other hoplites "wonder if Stelios will die" at the hands of the Captain, but Leonidas called an end to the beating—something the Captain appeared not to hear. Leonidas, enraged he wasn't listened to, leapt upon the Captain and beat him senseless. The young man, renamed Stumblios, was then told by Leonidas to pick up the unconscious Captain and carry him. Leonidas then punishes all the Spartans with "No food till journey's end," while the narrator comments "In *shame* ... we *march*" (Miller 2006, emphasis original). After camp was set up, Dilios, the story's narrator, told a tale of Leonidas's education in the Spartan *agoge* and how Leonidas embraced pain during his initiation period and survived the wild with no more than a long sharpened stick. It was with a stick that Leonidas killed the wolf that hunted him. With this feat Leonidas skinned the wolf, donned its fur and returned to Sparta a warrior and then king. Snyder's filmic narrative also incorporated this coming of age story as well (Snyder 2007).

Both narratives locate the indexical sign of pain at the center to speak of properly masculine warriors; men who are able to endure the furrows that mark the passing of the indexical sign of pain even as they are able to mete out such markings. A boy, then youth and finally a man who can stand and take blows and who can fall beneath the blows, but stand up again and ask for more, evinced the kind of masculinity the Spartan *agoge* inculcated in its male citizens. We are presented in the film and graphic novel with young flesh that is soft, sweet and unmarred which, through the process of becoming a man who exhibits *andreia* or the virtue of a warrior (Petterssen 1992, 42), is torn, bruised, and cut providing a geography of pain that indexically marks the growth of the boy into a Spartiate. He must, through a plethora of rites of passage (bare knuckle fights, lashing, and exposure), embrace the pain that both Miller and Snyder represent as the royal road to a super human masculine virility now lost in the distance past with ancient Sparta.

The indexical sign of pain is central to the construction of Spartan masculinity in the film and novel. Linked to the capacity to transcend and incorporate pain is a clarity of existence and an engagement with truth that is registered in the nakedness of the Spartan hoplite. Naked, his masculinity is exposed for all to see and if there was lack then this too would be exposed. Theron, unlike Leonidas, covers his body and he does not sport the crimson cloak, the mark of a Spartiate who has successfully completed his education. Lacking this cloak, and in Spartan terms, Theron is represented as a trembler; that is a male who failed in the Spartan system, in the *agoge* or the military. In

Theron, the viewer is presented with a Spartan political figure who has been bought, like the ephorate, by the Persians. Like the Persians, then, Theron wears too much clothing signifying his turn to the "orientalism" of Persia.

Naked, honest, and lacking deceit, the Spartan hoplite of the film and novel marched to the sound of the *diaulos* or double reed pipe, ritually played to lead the warriors to battle and possibly a beautiful death.[5] Lacking clothing and signs of material wealth, the Spartiate is free in the way other men, who are slaves to their passions and their gods, are not. The ephorate, represented as populated by disease-ridden monstrosities, clings to the "remnants of the old times, times prior to Lykourgos the law-giver" (Miller 2006). The Spartiatae, such as Leonidas and his 300, were free men who could not be awed by pain or deities.

Plutarch's Spartan, like Miller's and Snyder's, was also a masculinity lost to the depths of time. Although certainly Sparta continued to exist, as did its ritualized disciplinary educational system, the *agoge* in the time of Plutarch no longer produced the kind of heroic masculinity once evinced by Spartans like Leonidas, Agesilaus, and Lycurgus lamented Plutarch. These are the great kings of the once great Sparta lost to the depths of time. Sayings attributed to Spartans by Plutarch highlight some of the attributes of a masculinity he admired and considered proper to men. Agesilaus, for example, is presented as eschewing all items of comfort and sleeping in a regular tent among his men (Plutarch 1931a, *Apoph. Lac.* 2.18), and refusing rich foods. He is represented as saying, "It's quite inappropriate for those who profess true manly qualities to accept such delicacies. Things which attract slavish characters are alien to free men" (*Apoph. Lac.* 2.24). As with Miller and Snyder, Plutarch represented Spartan masculinity as raw, honest and lacking deceit. The Spartan warrior in his lack of apparel cannot conceal weakness and deception. Naked he is exposed to the eyes of all, and in this nakedness also signified honesty, truthfulness and non-duplicity; attributes Plutarch considered important to proper masculinity and something Spartan warriors displayed. This indifference to comfort and forthright engagement with the hardness of life Plutarch attributes to the laws of Lycurgus and the disciplinary educational system that focused on the making of warriors:

> Of reading and writing, they learned only enough to serve their turn; all the rest of their training was calculated to make them obey commands well, endure hardships, and conquer in battle. Therefore, as they grew in age, their bodily exercise was increased; their heads were close-clipped, and they were accustomed to going bare-foot, and to playing for the most part without clothes. When they were twelve years old, they no longer had tunics to wear,

received one cloak a year, had hard, dry flesh, and knew little of baths and ointments; only on certain days of the year, and few at that, did they indulge in such amenities.

(*Lyc.* 16.6)

Plutarch's Spartan's masculinity also includes references to freedom, but Plutarch's understanding of freedom takes slavery to be normative. And, although certainly Plutarch was aghast at the idea of the Krypteia and the murdering of helots and he also did not accept as unproblematic the enslavement of the Messenians, as both Miller and Snyder did; he does not, however, fully and utterly embraced the discourse of Spartan warriors as the only truly free men. Equally, Plutarch did not see a conflict between the strict obedience citizens owed to Sparta and their freedom in his texts. Instead, Plutarch locates freedom in obedience in his *bios* of Lycurgus:

> Wherefore, I for one am amazed at those who declare that the Lacedaemonians knew how to obey, but did not understand how to command, and quote with approval the story of King Theodosius, who, when someone said that Sparta was safe and secure because her kings knew how to command, replied: 'Nay, rather because her citizens know how to obey.' For men will not consent to obey those who have not the ability to rule, but obedience is a lesson to be learned from a commander. For a good leader makes good followers, and just as the final attainment of the art of horsemanship is to make a horse gentle and tractable, so it is the task of the science of government to implant obedience in men. And the Lacedaemonians implanted in the rest of the Greeks not only a willingness to obey, but a desire to be their followers and subjects. People did not send requests to them for ships, or money, or hoplites, but for a single Spartan commander; and when they got him, they treated him with honour and reverence.
>
> (*Lyc.* 30.3–5)

And, even as the Spartiatae were represented as obedient and yet truly free, they were also represented as pious; indeed, proper men are pious men who recognize and are obedient to proper authority. Plutarch commends the observance Sparta and Spartans paid to the deities and ritual. Unlike Miller's and Snyder's representation of Spartan masculinity, then, piety and not atheism, was the mark of the rational man. Plutarch wrote that:

> Agesilaus had now been nearly two years in the field, and much was said about him in the interior parts of Asia, and a wonderful opinion of his self-restraint, of his simplicity of life, and of his moderation, everywhere prevailed. For when he made a journey, he would take up his quarters in the most sacred precincts

by himself, thus making the gods overseers and witnesses of those acts which few men are permitted to see us perform.

(*Ages.* 14.1)

Plutarch also wrote that the two kings of Sparta, from the families of the Agaids and Eurypotids, both of whom trace their ancestry back to the sons of Heracles, the Heracleidae, were considered priests in the field and would sacrifice and if not the king then the seer who accompanied the kings into battle would make the offering (*Ages.* 6.5). In Plutarch's representation of Spartan masculinity obedience to authority, be it the laws of Lycurgus, Sparta and its political structure, and the deities, Apollo and Artemis-Ortheia, both of whom are represented as overseeing the lives of Sparta's next generation, are central.

Plutarch, again unlike Miller and Snyder, had no difficulty with the sexual aspects of the mentor relationship between adult male Spartiatae and Spartan boys once they were twelve years of age. He wrote in Lycurgus:

> When the boys reached this age, they were favoured with the society of lovers from among the reputable young men. The elderly men also kept close watch of them, coming more frequently to their places of exercise, and observing their contests of strength and wit, not cursorily, but with the idea that they were all in a sense the fathers and tutors and governors of all the boys. In this way, at every fitting time and in every place, the boy who went wrong had someone to admonish and chastise him.
>
> (*Lyc.* 17.1)

Plutarch, did, however, try to temper the pederasty by emphasizing Spartans like Lycurgus and Agesilaus appreciated the beauty of young boys, but taught them the ways of war rather than of love. Plutarch wrote that although Agesilaus was very tempted, he never gave into his desires (*Ages* 11.5 6). The issue, for Plutarch, however, was not heteronormativity; rather, properly masculine men should not be ruled by fear or love.

The Spartans' ritual use of pain is also represented in the writings of Plutarch. The indexical sign of pain is traced by furrows across the surface of the flesh via with the rod, whip, fist, and/or sword to mark the properly masculine Spartiate. Plutarch represents Agesilaus as one such Spartiate, as a warrior and king who put his men before himself as he did when, severely wounded, he refused rest until he was sure all the Spartan dead had been retrieved from the field of war (*Ages.* 19.1). In Plutarch's mythography endurance of pain signifies the intact masculinity of the Spartiate. *Lycurgus* is quite telling in this regard:

> The boys make such a serious matter of their stealing, that one of them, as the story goes, who was carrying concealed under his cloak a young fox which he had stolen, suffered the animal to tear out his bowels with its teeth and claws, and died rather than have his theft detected. And even this story gains credence from what their youths now endure, many of whom I have seen expiring under the lash at the altar of Artemis-Ortheia.
>
> (*Lyc.* 18.1)

Xenophon's mythography of Sparta and its manly warriors greatly influenced the work of Plutarch. Xenophon (430–354 BCE) lived during the period that Plutarch represented as the last years of the greatness of Sparta: it was during the reign of Agesilaus in 371 BCE that Messenia was lost to Sparta and its lands cut by half with potential threats to its polis on all its borders (Christien 2006, 176). Sparta had been soundly defeated at the battle of Luetra (371 BCE) by the Thebans, and Messenia and the helots had been liberated. Xenophon, however, does not discuss in any detail the helots of Sparta other than as a kind of people among others who are either serving Sparta in a military capacity or represented among those who were threatening Sparta. A slavery economy was normative of Greek warfare and warfare a frequent occurrence in the ancient world.

If warfare was common in the ancient world, then certainly the warrior was a common and necessary figure in the ancient world and in light of Sparta's militaristic turn, particularly so here. Xenophon, himself a soldier, respected the Spartan system of governance and disciplinary education. A noble himself, and having fought with Cyrus the Younger in Persia, Xenophon returned with the 10,000 Greeks who found themselves adrift in Persia upon Cyrus's death (401 BCE). He wrote of this event and journey home in his text *Anabasis*. It was during this arduous journey that Xenophon met and was befriended by Agesilaus, king of Sparta.

Xenophon's representation of Agesilaus is one of admiration for the king and for all things Spartan, particularly their capacity for warfare. The Spartan hoplite was an exquisite work of art; beautiful, graceful, strong, enduring, noble and obedient. Produced in through the disciplinary education system, and maintained by a militarily structured social organization, the Spartan male, as exemplified by Agesilaus, was the epitome of proper warrior masculinity:

> If line and rule are a noble discovery of man as aids to the production of good work, I think that the virtue of Agesilaus may well stand as a noble example for those to follow who wish to make moral goodness a habit. For who that imitates a pious, a just, a sober, a self-controlled man, can come to be

unrighteous, unjust, violent, wanton? In point of fact, Agesilaus prided himself less on reigning over others than on ruling himself, less on leading the people against their enemies than on guiding them all to virtue.

(*Ages.* 10.2)

The writing attributed to Xenophon repeatedly emphases self-control, moderation, modesty, and obedience as the scaffolding that supported Spartan masculinity. Engendered in the ritualized disciplinary education system, Spartan masculinity was a warrior masculinity that was necessary for the preservation of Sparta, not simply in its protective aspects, but equally to secure wealth for Sparta. Although certainly Xenophon emphasizes Lycurgus's rejection of wealth (*Const. Lac.* 7), Sparta nonetheless enriched it coffers with its warfare. And this kind of acquisition of wealth for the polis and those running it was not marked as problematic as this kind of wealth, and its attendant enslavement of subjugated peoples, was represented as the well-deserved spoils of victory.

In antithesis to the proper Spartiate in Xenophon's texts is the figure of what will officially be called the trembler by the first century BCE. In the Spartan system the masculinity of one who shrank from certain pain and possible death was called into serious question, and in light of this, wrote Xenophon, rightfully became a marked man: "For he [Lycurgus] believed, it seems, that enslavement, fraud, robbery, are crimes that injure only the victims of them; but the wicked man and the coward are traitors to the whole body politic. And so he had good reason, I think, for visiting their offences with the heaviest penalties" (*Const. Lac.* 10.6). Those who were improperly masculine faced significant social censure in the laws he attributed to Lycurgus, but in the representation of the operative quotidian of the Spartans, this censure did at times, wrote Plutarch, put the polis at risk insofar the population of the so-called tremblers was at times significantly greater than the Spartiatae raising the specter of sedation (*Ages.* 30).

Xenophon did not dwell on nakedness or even the dress of Spartan males other than to comment that it was simple for the boys who were in the disciplinary-educational systems and consisted of one robe and *chinton* for those under twelve and a *himation* for those older (Petterssen 1992, 81). Xenophon's Spartiatae were not represented as well-muscled, semi-naked men going into battle, while Plutarch related a tale wherein a young Spartiate, ran from his house with neither clothing nor armor and although he won the field and helped to prevent Sparta from being overrun, he was nonetheless fined for such an act (*Ages.* 34.5–8).

Xenophon's writings also represents Spartans and their kings as pious and attentive to their duties as priest and sacrificer. Xenophon wrote that

Agesilaus left the army to return to Sparta to participate in the Hyakinthia (*Ages.* 2.17), and conjectured "on the inspiring sight it would have been to watch Agesilaus and all his soldiers behind him returning garlanded from the gymnasium and dedicating their garlands to Artemis. For where men reverence the gods, train themselves in warfare and practise obedience, there you surely find high hopes abounding." (*Ages.* 1.27). It did not pay for any leader to be unmindful of the gods, and the kings of Sparta were mindful to pay respect to the deities. The kings of Sparta acted as priests of Zeus and offered sacrifice on behalf of the army and after a successful military campaign. At the time the Spartans spotted the opposing army, the king would sacrifice a goat, the soldiers put on wreaths and then began to sing the paean to Apollo marching to the rhythm of anapestic song (Petterssen 1992, 63).

Equally, according to Xenophon, the relations between the lover-mentor and beloved-mentee were properly non-sexual. The issue for Xenophon was not same-sex relations, but had more to do with the age gap when boys of the age of twelve entered into a relationship with an adult male:

> If someone, being himself an honest man, admired a boy's soul and tried to make of him an ideal friend without reproach and to associate with him, he [Lycurgus] approved, and believed in the excellence of this kind of training. But if it was clear that the attraction lay in the boy's outward beauty, he banned the connexion as an abomination; and thus he caused lovers to abstain from boys no less than parents abstain from sexual intercourse with their children and brothers and sisters with each other.
>
> (*Const. Lac.* 2.13)

For Xenophon, the proper man never succumbed to desire of any kind as this signified weakness (*Ages.* 5.4–7).

Pain also figures in Xenophon's mythography of Spartan masculinity. Xenophon presents a disciplinary educational system wherein endurance of pain is central to the construction of Spartan warrior masculinity:

> [T]he Spartans chastise those who get caught for stealing badly. He [Lycurgus] made it a point of honour to steal as many cheeses as possible [from the altar of Artemis-Ortheia], but appointed others to scourge the thieves, meaning to show thereby that by enduring pain for a short time one may win lasting fame and felicity.
>
> (*Const. Lac.* 2. 8–9)

In Xenophon's text the indexical sign of pain, furrows left by fist, lash, or sickle, is central to the construction of Spartan warrior masculinity.

Ritual and the Altar of Ortheia

The three significant Spartan festivals, the Hyakinthia, the Gymnopaidiai, and the Karneia, Petterssen argues, are parts of a ritual cycle that marks a rite of passage for males in Sparta. Drawing on Arnold van Gennep's tripartite structure of separation, liminality and integration he argues that the Hyakinthia represented the rite of separation, the gymnopaidiai the rite of liminality and the Karneia the rite of integration bringing the males back into the community with a new status, that of a warrior (Petterssen 1992, 78). The Hyakinthia (age classes 7-19; 20-29 years old) marked the death of Apollo's young lover, killed by him in accident with a discus. The first segment of the festival is somber and marks the death of Hyakinthos, who is lost to Apollo. Equally, this kind of loss is experienced by the parents of the boys who are removed from their families and become a herd of boys who share an age group and must learn to survive. The gymnopaidiai (age classes 7-19; 20-29; 30-59; 60+ years old), he argued, represented a period of liminality, wherein there were tests of endurance, and it was at this time, Petterssen argued, the ordeal of cheese stealing (age class 14-17 yrs. old), later in the Roman period the diamastigosis or whipping on the altar of Artemis-Ortheia, and the Krypteia (age class 18-19 years old), or the so-called helot hunt, occurred. The military festival of the Karneia, honoring Apollo Karneios (Ram), completed the ritual cycle and the boys, now men (21-29; 30+ years old), became Sparta's warriors (Pettersson 1992, 89) The ritual cycle did not have well-drawn lines within the festivals or between them in terms of activities related to rites and tended to include all age classes in each festival (ibid.).

Having been removed from their families during the Hyakinthia and now living among each other and with other male Spartans of all ages, the gymnopaidiai, the next festival, emphasized the liminal space and time[6] that the boys occupied and served as part of the process of transforming the child into an adult, the boy into man, and the potential warrior to the Spartiate, the Spartan warrior-citizen, in the ritualized disciplinary educational system called the *agoge*. And, at the center of the transformation, the means by which it was largely achieved, was pain, endured and inflicted, marking the passage. Young boys sang in choir and performed dances naked and in the heat of the sun, they competed with each other and with all males of other age classes in choral song, music and dance, all of which were offerings to Apollo Pythaeus, Artemis, and Leto whose statues viewed the performances while they danced the *gymnopaidike orkhesis*. Petterssen (1992, 47) has argued that this kind of performance before the deities Apollo, Artemis and Leto—the former two linked to children and youth (Leto was their mother)—is highly suggestive of initiation.[7]

The ball-boxing game, referred to as the *Spairomachiai*, was also agonistic in form and players were said to strike each other with sticks and fists during the game. A primary aspect of the game was the delivery and reception of pain marking victors from losers. The game has been linked to Gymnopaidiai festival, and considering the agonistic nature of the festival in general it certainly seems possible. The welt from the stick is the indexical sign of pain signifying a transition from boy to warrior. Equally, the burn and heat from the sun while performing or cracked and rent bare feet of unshod youth signified the passage of pain and the willingness to engage it. As Xenophon wrote, "...by enduring pain for a short time one may win lasting fame and felicity" (*Const. Lac.* 2.9).

In his work Petterssen connected the thrashing/flogging at the Altar of Ortheia and the Krypteia with the Gymnopaidiai arguing that they were tests of endurance (1992, 45), which clearly they were, but that is not the only requirement of the test. Pain for the sake of pain and as an indexical sign that left its mark on the bodies and minds of all the participants was absolutely central to the rite. Even Artemis participated in the meeting out of pain in that her *xoanon*, held by her priest, was said to grow heavier if the whipping at her altar was not vigorous enough (ibid., 46). The rite of the theft of the cheese from Artemis-Ortheia's altar required that the boys steal as much cheese as they could in the face of brutal lashes rained down upon them by the older youth who must protect the altar and its cheese. The rite is without a doubt agonistic and clearly linked to warfare: a warfare enacted by both groups in their struggle to gain or save the cheese. In the game of war pain was the central signifier marking the acquisition of proper Spartan warrior masculinity. Linked to the cheese agon at the altar of Ortheia was the later flagellation or the *diamastigosis* that Plutarch indicated he witnessed. This version of the rite reflects a clearer statement of enduring pain, insofar as some youths, Plutarch related, died under the lash (*Lyc.* 18.1).

The rite of the Krypteia, or the so-called helot-hunting, was said by a number of ancient authors to have been practiced by the Spartans. Plutarch, against Plato and Aristotle, denied that Lycurgus could have come up with such an abominable practice and instead proposed that the practice emerged after the earthquake (369 BCE) and when the helots and Messenians revolted (369 BCE) (*Lyc.* 28.6). Petterssen suggests that the ritual of the Krypteia occurred just prior to young men entering the army, that is, at eighteen to nineteen years of age. Divest of all clothing, weaponless, and without allies, the soon-to-be hoplite warrior must survive, some say for a year, and during this time remain unseen while hunting helots on the roads (Petterssen 1992, 45). Although there is lack of clarity around the practice of helot-hunting and its inclusion in the Krypteia, or how long ritualized helot-hunting was practiced in Sparta, it certainly would be a strong ritualized practice that inculcated in youth obedience to inflict pain and bring about death following orders given by recognized authorities (Aristotle in Ducat 2006b, 284). Pain, again, acts as an indexical sign that marks the next transition, which was membership in the army. The Krypteia, then, is the other side of the play of pain in the games of war, but now rather than simply enduring pain, the effort was to also inflict it. Once this final rite was completed and the lesson learned; that is, to inflict pain in an instant and to do so without question, the budding hoplite was allowed to grow his hair long and was given a bronze shield, weapons and a red cloak; red because it was considered a masculine color (Xenophon, *Const. Lac.* 11.4).

In both Miller and Snyder's mythography Leonidas is represented during the period of the Krypteia wherein he is presented as cold and threatened by a wolf in the mountains around Sparta. He slays the animal and takes his skin, which provided Leonidas with warmth. The reader and viewer are provided a narrative of a direct and resourceful young Leonidas who will be a direct and resourceful mature king. There is no reference to the hunting of helots, or even to helots in general. In shots of the countryside we see tall stands of golden wheat representing agricultural wealth and the home of Sparta, but nary a helot is in sight. Even though the reader/viewer is aware that Leonidas has claimed war as the only profession of the proper Spartiate, we are not invited to ask how Spartans feed and clothe themselves if "free" Spartans do not labor like "slaves" but perform their natural labor; war (and for women giving birth to warriors). Both Miller and Snyder are white Americans and as such should be aware of the cost of ignoring slavery.

Ortheia (Artemis) Altar

The altar of Ortheia appeared to have been at the center of a number of festivals and rites in Sparta. Found in the sanctuary are deposits as early as the tenth century BCE and they continued until circa 350 CE. The altar with temonos were the earliest structures over which was built the archaic altar, then the Greek altar in circa 550 BCE along with the first rough temple, which was rebuilt in the second century CE. Found at the earliest level were geometric pottery shards and through the levels were found bronze, bone, ivory, lead and iron objects, and figurines. Included as well were terracotta masks. These masks came in a number of kinds: the smoothed-faced hero and the contorted and deeply etched Gorgon, Satyr and Furrowed Grotesque. Also found are stelai with impressions of sickles and the names of youthful victors of the *agōnes*, choral, dance, and hunting competitions enacted at or near the altar. Also found were sickles presumably dedicated by the ritual participants. A Roman theatre was added to the site in the second century CE and the temonos of the area expanded in the third century CE, while the altar was rebuilt by the Romans for the last time circa 250 CE (Bosanquet et al. 1906, 61). The continued development of the sanctuary indicates that the altar of Ortheia, and then Artemis-Ortheia, was an important site for Spartan ritual engagement, and particularly a site for ritual with regard to children, male and female, and their process toward adulthood. It was here that the performance of gender, significantly masculine gender, was enacted under the eyes of all in the agonistic theatre of becoming a warrior in ancient Sparta.

The altar of Ortheia, at the center of the sanctuary, played a significant role in the *agōnes*, but in particular the cheese-stealing rite and then later the rite of flagellation that Plutarch referenced in a number of his writings:

> The boys in Sparta were lashed with whips during the entire day at the altar of Artemis-Ortheia, frequently to the point of death, and they bravely endured this, cheerful and proud, vying with one another for the supremacy as to which one of them [p. 445] could endure being beaten for the longer time and the greater number of blows. And the one who was victorious was held in especial repute. This competition is called "The Flagellation," and it takes place each year.
>
> (Plutarch 1931b, *Inst.* 40)

Standing nearby was the female priest who held the *xoanon* of Artemis-Ortheia and if the blows too light, then the *xoanon* was said to grow heavier indicating the deity's displeasure. As the event and the blood were meant for her pleasure, her displeasure was taken seriously especially by the Spartans whose piety was commented upon by ancient authors like Plutarch and Xenophon.

The *diamastigosis* drew spectators every year and ancient authors speculated as to its origins. Pausanias, the second century CE traveler-historian, upon visiting the site wrote that the *xoanon*, of Ortheia had been causing calamities ever since it was found. The wooden image, Pausanias relates, was stolen from the Tauric land by Orestes and Iphigenia, and when found by the great-great-great-grandsons of Agis I (ninth and eighth centuries BCE) caused madness, rage and brought about death. An oracle was sent and the Spartans were told, according to Pausanias, "that they should stain the altar with human blood":

> He used to be sacrificed upon whomsoever the lot fell, but Lycurgus changed the custom to a scourging of the lads, and so in this way the altar is stained with human blood. By them stands the priestess, holding the wooden image.

Now it is small and light, but if ever the scourgers spare the lash because of a lad's beauty or high rank, then at once the priestess finds the image grow so heavy that she can hardly carry it. She lays the blame on the scourgers, and says that it is their fault that she is being weighed down. So the image ever since the sacrifices in the Tauric land keeps its fondness for human blood.
(Pausanias 3.16.10–11)

In Pausanias's telling, the sanctuary and altar come into being in order to deflect the wrath of the Artemis-Ortheia. In ancient Greek myth both Orestes and Iphigenia were closely linked to Artemis and Apollo.[8] The two fled Tauris, where Iphigenia served as priest to Artemis, and returned to Sparta with the *xoanon* of Artemis, having stolen it from her temple. In Pausanias's narrative, then, the youths Iphigenia and Orestes are linked to Artemis and Apollo in ritualistic actions that are saturated with blood, and haunted by illicit sex, murder, matricide and human sacrifice. This is the miasma associated with the *xoanon* that must be, wrote Paussanias, assuaged with the blood of male youths, enduring, sometimes unto death, the whip that tore their flesh leaving in its wake red-glistening tears incised upon the naked backs, buttocks, and legs of the boys who would become warriors at the altar of Artemis-Ortheia.

Conclusion

The sanctuary and altar of Artemis-Ortheia is the final discursive threat examined that represents the tapestry of Spartan masculinity. The altar itself and the deity, Artemis-Ortheia, were part of this process of masculation or bringing into a state of masculinity as defined by the group. In Pausanias, the narrative of the wooden statue locates *xoanon* as prior to and the reason for the sanctuary, as were the lashings delivered at the altar. In Xenophon, however, we have a different narrative: instead youths strategized against each other in an agon over cheese at the altar. The weaponless younger youth faced the older youth who with lashes and/or rods struck them as they endeavored to steal the cheese enduring a rain of vicious blows. Both groups were ensconced within the *agoge*, and this act of theft, like the later ritual lashing, required one embrace pain, either in its reception or its delivery. Pain was an indexical sign that, like tree rings, marked the growth of the boy into a proper Spartiate: that is, one who received pain as easily as he delivered it.

Both Plutarch and Xenophon reference the altar of Artemis-Ortheia in their mythographies of Spartan masculinities and both associate the altar with the *agoge*; that is the ritually framed disciplinary-education system in Sparta. The narrative of the whipping acts a touchstone that grounds their mythographies in ancient Spartan ritualistic practices instituted by Lycurgus is manifested particularly in the *agoge*. Such ritual is represented as the bedrock of Spartan masculinity. When Spartan males deviated from this, they were seen to have deviated from their true natures and as such joined the class of tremblers. Pain acted as the center of the truth of Spartan masculinity and the incised flesh of boys marked their passage into what both Xenophon and Plutarch considered to be heroic warriors. Both considered the ravishment, slaughter, and enslavement of populations to be a matter of course, while warriors-soldiers fit into this matter of course. Sparta was not only a defensive polis, it was often on the offensive and if Spartan warriors stood strong at Thermopylae, other conflicts they were regularly engaged in were to secure wealth, particularly when they lost their base of wealth when the helots and others of Messenia ended Spartan domination. Many consider the Krypteia to have emerged at this time when Sparta went on the defensive surrounded as they were by enemies. Attacking other Greeks such as the Thebans meant not merely a battlefield conflict but also included the ravagement of the peoples in and near the conflict if the winners happen to be the attackers. Kathy Gaca's study of ancient warfare and the military strategy of ravishment of the population as necessary to victory makes very clear the kind of anguish and pain that was inflicted by hoplites (Gaca 2015). Those who were old faced "mocking torment" which amounted to being tortured to death for the amusement of warriors. In some cases all males were put to death, in others young boys were taken as slaves, and were often publicly raped. Females not considered useful as plunder died via lethal gang rape, while females considered viable plunder endured "controlled access rape," that is she became the property of the soldier who then used and/or sold her as he saw fit (ibid., 278–281). This ravishment, of course, was not just enacted by Spartans warriors, but also by other Greek armies, who took the Spartans to be the best of warriors. Ideally, then, no quarter was to be given by proper warriors.

In the mythographies of Xenophon and Plutarch, the altar of Artemis-Ortheia located in its marshy and liminal geographical space, served to anchor their narratives of Spartan masculinity in the mystery of devotion to Artemis-Ortheia evidenced in the pain and blood given over to her. Jean-Pierre Vernant wrote that Artemis Kourotrophos supervised the training of male youths in the hunt, a practice linked to warfare in the ancient world. Hunting and warfare combined, wrote R. Lomis, "to raise mold, educate, and discipline future soldiers from the cradle to the battlefield" (in Zeitlin 1991, 243) and, of course, to the grave. Artemis, like her brother Apollo, was a deity that afflicted youth even as she protected them. Apollo loved Hyakinthos and yet also killed him. Artemis equally demanded the life of Iphigenia for her father's mistake. And regardless that Artemis saved Iphigenia from death, she doomed her to participate in the sacrifice of fellow Hellenes should they happen upon the temple (Euripides 1938, 1.1–40). Both Artemis and Apollo brought affliction with their care.

The ancient world continues to fascinate people, and Frank Miller and Zack Snyder are two such people. Miller's rendition of Spartan masculinities, like Snyder's, revels in the pain locating the emergence of proper masculinity in the test of the Krypteia, although a wolf rather than an unaware helot was the adversary. Miller's proper Spartans, the *hippeis* (Christien 2006, 175–176), or the 300 Spartan hoplite soldiers who acted as the king's chosen men, endured, like their king, the elements and hardships of warfare and stood strong against the overwhelming odds of the overdressed and effeminate Persians, a representation of the Persians Snyder takes to the monstrous in his film.

As with any gender ideology played out in binaries, evident in the first thread of the mythic tapestry of Spartan masculinity and carried forward to Snyder's film, the position of the same, ipseity, is given positive value and the position of the other, alterity, negative value. The failed masculine trembler stands in contrast to the successful masculine warrior; as does the coward to the brave, the feminine to the masculine, the young to the mature, the human to the deity, the orient to the occident, the prey to the hunter and the civilian to the warrior. The sign by which value was indexed is pain. To receive pain, and indeed embrace it, as both Snyder and Miller have Leonidas and his 300 do, and to impart gut-wrenching pain building meters-high walls with dead bodies, as presented in the film and graphic novel, make pain central to their constructions of masculinities. Like Plutarch, Xenophon, and the ritual actors at the altar of Artemis-Ortheia, pain is the indexical sign that is integral to the myth of the making of the Spartan warrior: an ideal of warriorhood found in the pages of our stories, past and present, about ancient Sparta. But even as we gaze in admiration of the warrior's ability to endure pain, we ignore how the boy-child got there and the pain he inscribes on the flesh of others—the hero mask conceals the demon inside.

Pain appears to have an interesting role as an indexical sign in the narratives and mythographies that relate the story of the human's relationship with deity. In ancient Sparta the affliction of Artemis-Ortheia was paid for with the blood of its male young. The idea of a god afflicting a human is certainly not new and certainly not only found in ancient Greece. Indeed the engagement with icons in modern rural Greece associated with Fire Walking is one whereby the saints, Constantine and his mother Helena (we could easily substitute Menelaus and Helen), afflict their chosen until such time as they take up the road of the saint (Danforth 1989). The deity and/or its emissaries such as heroes like Hyakinthos, Orestes, and Iphigenia, or saints such as Constantine, manifest their relationships in the flesh via the indexical sign pain. It is pain that marks the pathway to deity securing the deflection of affliction and establishing a significant relationship with deity, and in other cases or in association with the first, the intimate dance with pain is seized upon in order to place one's feet upon the mystical path to the realm of the big Other. Against Elaine Scarry, then, pain does not escape language, indeed it is a particular script that is incised and made meaningful in the flesh.

Chapter 4

Penetrating the Body of the Masculine Other
White Masculinity, War, and Ritualized Torture

Introduction

My effort in this chapter is to develop a discussion concerning gendering and racializing in the application of the indexical sign of pain. To do this I engage the events at Abu Ghraib that captured on camera what appears to be the ritualized torture and humiliation of a number of Iraqi prisoners. It is my intention to make visible the semiotic link between the indexical sign of pain, white US masculinity, and race in the application of torture to "soften up" the bodies of prisoners before, during and after interrogation at Abu Ghraib in 2003. By developing a semiotics of pain, or how pain signifies, in this case the femininity and defeat of the Islamic other, I wish to disrupt how pain is represented as pure and desocialized experience and exempt from such categories as gender, race, geopolitical location, and class, and furthermore to speak to the deleterious outcomes from the intersection of gender, race, and pain in the neocolonial context of the so-called "war on terror."

Context and Problem

There is no doubt that what occurred on September 11, 2001—the penetration of New York's World Trade Center twin towers by two hijacked commercial aircraft—has been vividly etched onto the imaginations of the majority of Americans (and people in other countries), and certainly has shaped the international presence of the United States. The images of the planes slicing their way through glass, metal, and cement like a knife through butter flashed across televisions around the globe. CNN, filming this event, ran a caption underneath proclaiming, "Breaking News: America under Attack." Shortly, as many of us who watched on our televisions recall, first the south tower and then the north tower collapsed, sending tremors across the New York cityscape and metaphorically around the globe. The images of aggressing and collapsing can signify many things, and among these, and important for this paper, were the vulnerability of the US Empire and a return of the repressed: the racialized and feminized heathen "other" of the Christian/

Jewish-colonialist fantasy who threatens order with chaos. The powerful bastion of economic, legal, and political power, the World Trade Center, was not invulnerable and had been shattered and penetrated, the final outcome of which was the rapid collapse of the twin towers.

Terrorism, although certainly not new to the US Empire, was something that other countries had to deal with, regardless of an earlier bombing of the World Trade Center in 1993. Terrorism as a concept although of concern in the 1990s in the United States was not fully exploited by the Reagan presidency and so the 1993 assault of the towers did not galvanize the US into a "war on terror": that would come later during the regime of George W. Bush and Dick Cheney after the events of September 11, 2001.

Refracted through a medium of xenophobia, at least in the Eurowest, terrorism is the fear of unknown assailants intent upon bringing about fear, chaos, mayhem, and death within a social body. They are imaged to penetrate the social body and in doing so make visible its "bodily" gaps that are vulnerable to (sexual) assault: To be sexually assaulted is to be feminized. These unknown assailants—dark, mysterious, faceless, militarized, fanatical, and non-Western—are seen to signify as a general threat emergent from "third world"[1] locations, in particular the Middle East, in the conceptualization of terrorism in the United States and the Eurowest in general. It does not matter that acts of terrorism also occur with great regularity in non-Eurowestern countries, as the coordinated attacks in Mumbai in November 2008 and the direct terrorizing of Gazian Palestinians by the Israeli government beginning late December 2008 and ending mid-January 2009 made apparent. Such places are outside of the Eurowest (even as they are inside).

Terrorism, and its constant and ubiquitous effects, loomed large in the imagined communities (Anderson 2006) of the United States and with it came the belief that protection from such attacks was required at all costs. The constant ramping up of fear of an external and continuous menace "softened up" the citizen body making it much more amenable to the use of torture; newly partnered with terrorism but certainly having been partnered in the past with militarism, law, medicine, and religion (Wisnewski 2010, 16–48). As Michel Foucault has written:

> The term "penal torture" does not cover any corporal punishment: it is a differentiated production of pain, an organized ritual for the marking of victims and the expression of the power that punishes; not the expression of a legal system driven to exasperation and, forgetting its principles, losing all restraint. In the "excesses" of torture, a whole economy of power is invested.
>
> (Foucault 1979, 34–35)

Torture is a process of intentionally inflicting pain in another living being for some purpose, often said to be the need for information, although torture used to acquire information has been demonstrated to be ineffectual and unreliable in the past and in the present (Rios and Mischkowski 2019, 934).[2] Torture is also used to alter a person, to break them down so that they may be rebuilt by the torturer or for the pleasure, often sexual, of the torturer (Carter 1990). Torture is also used to interrogate, punish, and demoralize the enemy other who represents a threat to the state. Although referring to the "criminal," the insight works equally well with the so-called terrorist:

> The fact that the crime and the punishment were related and bound up in the form of atrocity [such as terrorism] was not the result of some obscurely accepted law of retaliation. It was the effect, in the rites of punishment, of a certain mechanism of power: of a power that not only did not hesitate to exert itself directly on the bodies, but was exalted and strengthened by its visible manifestations ...
>
> (Foucault 1979, 57)

Jeremy Wisnewski (2010, 7-8) lists six different kinds of torture: judicial, punitive, interrogational, dehumanizing, terroristic/deterrent and sadistic, although most of these overlap in some fashion or another. Instruments of torture are legion, reflecting technologies of different historical periods. In the early modern period of France, the torture of a witch or sorcerer (the narrative of witchcraft was highly gendered) consisted of several technologies of torture, one being the *brodequins* (boots) wherein wooden planks were tied around the legs of the person between which, legs and planks, wedges were lodged. The number of wedges used was related to the crime. When severely applied leg bones were shattered as in the case of the priest Urbain Grandier charged with sorcery in sixteenth century Loudun (Juschka 2009, 104). At the center of torture is the fully and wholly embodied self, a self utterly embodied and who must passively, having been restrained, accept the painful inscriptions on and to their body. All the while, the tortured must accept the responsibility for the pain as it is their own actions that have compelled the torturers to etch pain into their bodies, while it is their body that succumbed to the pain (Wisnewski 2010, 38-39; Scarry 1985, 35-36).

Pain effected through torture is at the center of this paper, while the site of torture this chapter engages is Abu Ghraib drawing upon the pictures that exposed the "softening up" of prisoners (under what has been named Standard Operating Procedures) in preparation for interrogation, and written documents recording further torture and death in the interrogation room.[3] As

I watched the unfolding of the story of Abu Ghraib in mainstream and alternative media, I was made uncomfortable with the voyeurism of the media, even as they condemned the pictures they flashed across television and computer screens around the globe. It wasn't so much the display of these images, since I think an historical record must be put in place, but the way the images were displayed often with little analysis, other than moral outrage, to the point of making more pornographic what was already pornographic.[4] In the presentation of these images there was little effort to understand how xenophobia, homophobia, ideologies of masculinity, and racism were integral to the actions of the military police personnel (seen in the pictures), the military (among others Major General Michael Dunlavey and Major General Geoffrey Miller), lawyers (among others Alberto Gonzales, John Yoo and Jay Bybee), government officials such as Donald Rumsfeld, George W. Bush, Dick Cheney, the media, and many who had, under the rationale of self-defense agreed to inscribe pain on the bodies of those taken as a means to penetrate the bodies and minds of the "other"; much as the twin towers had been penetrated.

To Be or Not to Be: Penetrated and Penetrator

Two aspects of torture must be adhered to in order that the monstrosity of the act not make monsters of those intent upon using it. Firstly, it must be secret or at least kept from the general population and removed from court intervention (Greenberg and Dratel 2005, xxi–xxii; Foucault 1979, 35). When torture could no longer be legitimately used as a domestic juridical tool or as a military tool in armed conflicts because of the Universal Declaration of Human Rights, the International Covenant on Civil and Political Rights, the Convention against Torture, and international humanitarian law in line with the Geneva Conventions, its deployment needed to be in space that was and was not legally defined as US space; in other words liminal space such as Guantánamo Bay or Abu Ghraib where neither the law nor the light of shame could bring a halt to practices of torture.[5] Public torture was a thing of the past and made illegal while governments openly eschewed the practice of torture as it signified barbarity and irrationality. Therefore, in light of the problem of publicly engaging in the practice of torture, it must be kept secret, or at least be a public secret.[6] Furthermore, as Lisa Silverman comments, "[i]n the modern world, torture is secret because of the contemporary conviction that it is only testimony that is given voluntarily that is true" (2001, 89).

Secondly, torture cannot appear to be applied willy-nilly: it must be encircled in such a way as to inhibit its spilling over spreading beyond the space of its application. Toward this end, torture is rationalized by the rules of its application (Rejali 2007, 446–479), while its application is enclosed by a rite of pain. The ritual enclosing of torture provides a (illusory) sense of control and, furthermore, the inscription of pain on the body can be deemed sane rather than insane: ritualization rationalizes torture so that it is but a tool rather than the sadistic actions of a crazed human. Equally, torture encapsulated by ritual provides epistemological surety that torture is a means to something greater than pain (and death) demarcating the real and imagined space between those who torture and those who are tortured. As for those participants of the ritual of torture, such as medical personnel who do not engage in the practice of torture but may be present for its *actus reus* they mark the circumference of the circle of pain between the so-called rational world and the irrational world of torture. The rite of torture allowed for a professional deployment of the indexical sign of pain as one of an arsenal of weapons, all while differentiating it from out and out sadism. But this differentiation is just an illusion:

> The state endorses torture for either intimidation or information. Once it does so, the incentives are such that torture "is carried out with positive probability"—regardless of the type of torturer. Even professionals succumb to the pressure to torture regardless. When the purpose is intimidation, "All types of torturers will behave sadistically.
>
> (Rejali 2007, 455)

Pain, as deployed in torture and torture as the ritual application of pain (clearly evinced in legalized and judicial use of torture throughout human history), is a means by which to penetrate the body of the "other" marked as enemy, traitor, witch, heretic, slave, and in this instance, the Middle Eastern/Islamic other. The body of the tortured is the place of penetration wherein the body is *opened* so that the "truth," whatever that truth, can be exposed. That truth may be proposed to be secrets that need to be ferreted out to give an advantage to the torturers; but often it is another truth that is sought: the bodies opened under torture are bodies that through having been penetrated reveal the feminine that is the nature of the male/masculine other. For example, interrogation technique nine, "Pride and Ego Down," is meant to demoralize a detainee by attacking the ego. In numerous instances at Abu Ghraib, female undergarments were given to detainees to wear on, or were placed over, their heads whereupon they were paraded around and jeered at by US soldiers (Greenberg and Dratel 2005, 392-393). Having to abide humiliation and torture, in the masculine sexual fantasy playing out in these so-called dark sites, the Iraqi male detainees signified as feminine and as defined within the white, US, seemingly heterosexual, military masculinity as a masculinity that cannot or should not be penetrated even under torture.⁷ The rules and applications of torture at Abu Ghraib were based upon "Survival, Evasion, Resistance, and Escape" (SERE), "a program designed to train US military personnel to withstand interrogation by enemy captors" (Jaffer and Singh 2007, 4–5). Those men (and women) who succumbed to torture either by breaking or dying signified their lack of proper (white, US, heterosexual, and warrior) masculinity.

US (Military) Masculinities

The dominant masculinity in the United States is signified by three important aspects that are consequential for this chapter: impenetrability, whiteness (understood as non-racialized) and Protestant Christianity. Proper masculinity is from the outset staunchly heterosexual, which in its current formation means that men are penetrators (active) and women are penetrated (passive) even if some of the soldiers should be female. Pierre Bourdieu has written that:

> Penetration, especially when performed on a man, is one of the affirmations of the *libido dominandi* that is never entirely absent from the masculine libido. It is known that in a number of societies homosexual possession is conceived as a manifestation of 'power', an act of domination (performed as such, in some cases, in order to assert superiority by 'feminizing' the other) ... It can be understood that from this point of view, which links sexuality and power,⁸ the worst humiliation for a man is to be turned into a woman.
> (Bourdieu 2001, 21–22)

Men who are penetrated, literally or symbolically, in this frame are not properly masculine and therefore are not men. They may have the bodies and voices of men (although if they lack English then certainly their speech is feminine "babble" or non-authoritative speech much as non-human animals), but lack the manliness that would signify that they are "real" men. Indeed, SERE training, "administered by the Joint Personnel Recovery Agency ('JPRA') at Fort Belvoir, Virginia," was said to have "deliberately humiliated, subjected to stress positions, forced to exercise to the point of exhaustion, and subjected to various forms of psychological duress" selected military personnel, "all to prepare them for the possibility of abuse and torture by foreign intelligence services" (Jaffer and Singh 2007, 5). As in ancient Athens, true men could keep silent "even under torture" (Herodotus *Persian Wars*, 8.110 in DuBois 1991, 25).

Properly masculine men do not succumb to torture. Proper men's flesh might be physically penetrated, but that which marked them as men in the Eurowest, their minds, are not. They were trained to adhere to masculine domination by resisting being dominated by other men (even more so by women) and trained not to break when their flesh is excised by the passage of pain under torture. To succumb to pain is to be absolutely penetrated and thereby feminized. Men who did (do) not succumb to pain were seen as intrinsically masculine lacking either feminine or queer tendencies and therefore properly masculine.

In the racialized context of the US, proper masculinity is a non-raced masculinity, while non-racialized masculinity defaults to white operating as unmarked. There are of course other masculinities in the United States (Black, Indigenous, Latino, and so forth), but these are marked by race and therefore deemed problematic to greater and lesser degrees. Black and Latino masculinities are often represented as a hypermasculinity insofar as they are seen as excessive masculinities: black masculinity is too aggressive both physically and sexually leading to criminal activity, hence the over-representation of black men in the US prison system, and Latino masculinity too male oriented so that homosexuality is seen as a potential threat hidden in this kind of masculinity. Race linked to and definitive of the kind of purported masculinity ensures that said masculinity is easily representable as problematic if not aberrant.[9]

A broad-based Protestant Christianity further contributes to the construction of a proper US masculinity. The Protestant Christianity engaged is not a specific form such as Methodist, Baptist, Episcopalian, and the like; rather it is an abstracted US Christianity definable in some measure by what it is not. Therefore it is not highly emotive as in Black US Baptist Churches nor is it dogmatic and oriented toward literalism as seen with the Southern Baptist Convention; rather, it is a diluted and broad-spectrum Protestantism,[10] something that might be seen to lean toward I. E. Bailey's (1997) concept of implicit religion or Max Weber's "ascetic Protestantism" (2001, xiii).

Raising Weber allows also for the introduction of capitalism, or at least its spirit, and brings to mind important defining aspects of the heroic capitalist who is normatively white and masculine: hard working, successful, determined, humorless, and morally righteous. This "ascetic Protestantism" works in tandem with whiteness, which refers us to the notion of those unmarked by race in a racist social body, and a properly sealed or impenetrable masculinity referring us to the proper positioning of femininity as different from and indeed oppositional[11] to masculinity. The class operative in this ascetic Protestantism is bourgeoisie so that the good life is depicted as owning a home (with wife and children as "he" is properly heterosexual), car or cars, money for trips, desired goods, and a comfortable retirement. What the good life looks like for Christian women is to have a home, kids, and husband. To acquire the good life requires competitiveness, toughness, single-mindedness, conviction, self-sacrifice, (tempered) loyalty, and a sense of camaraderie. These categories are already highly coded by our social systems, but linked to an overtly non-raced, impenetrable (heterosexual), middle-class masculine ideal, the magnitude of their signification increases. "Ascetic Protestantism," whiteness, and an impenetrable masculinity come together to form the ideal of the manly man, a dominant ideal of the masculine operative in the United States (and certainly aspects of this ideal can be found throughout the Eurowest). There are of course variations of this ideal, but its central markers of the absence of race, impenetrability, conviction, toughness, righteousness, and competitiveness (Juschka 2009, 86–88) tend to be present.

The instability of the social categories of masculinities, femininities (gender ideology), race and class, and the instability of borders between these categories requires that they be constantly shored up, as Judith Butler has so astutely argued (see Butler 1999, 2003, 2004). This shoring up includes active and hostile defense, particularly when understood to be under threat and certainly the destruction of the twin towers in 2001 was a very real threat. In the face of such an attack and in the military response to this, seen in the United States' war on terror culminated in the invasion of Iraq, US masculinity was in need of vigorous defense, even if it should mean the distorted construction and violent penetration and annihilation of the feminized other who had threatened to contaminate US masculinity. US masculinity must reassert its dominance on the global stage. The manly nation of United States and its properly manly men were not "namby pambies."

If this is a generic US masculinity, how does US militarized masculinity intersect with it? US generic masculinity (white and Protestant) is found wanting once young men and women enter their military training period, and this too soft masculinity must be shored up with a more "robust" masculinity, one that will produce "strong" (however strong is defined), but obedient soldiers. Independence of thought, at least among enlisted personnel, must be squelched, while discipline and respect for authority deployed through hierarchical structures normative to the military must be engendered. As Cynthia Enloe has convincingly argued, the militarized version of the US masculine ideal is a central aspect in the ideology of militarism and the sociopolitical process of militarization (2004, 219). Furthermore, the boundary between militarism and civilian masculinities in the United States is amorphous enough that telling them apart is often difficult. There is a tendency to think that there is a natural and normative link between masculinity and militarism, and this tendency is reinforced daily in media, war museums, film, story, image, speech; the list is endless. Enloe writes that "men are on most war museums' center stage because war is imagined to be a masculinized process ..." (2004, 196).

Legal, Political, and Military Discourses on Torture

The efforts by the hegemonic parties involved to normalize the use of torture in the United States involved producing a number of discourses by which to engage torture. In US popular culture, for example, Fox's television series *24* (first aired November 6, 2001, and running eight seasons) and *The Passion of the Christ* (2004, co-written, produced, and directed by Mel Gibson[12]) jump to mind. In *24* pain is etched on the body with torture used to force the "truth" from the bodies of the so-called terrorists who are seen to succumb to pain and provide good "intel" and "actionable intelligence."[13] Indeed, in season four torture was presented as necessary and unavoidable if men (properly masculine US men) were to save their nation. In *The Passion*, however, we see a different signification of the inscription of the indexical sign of pain; it is the means by which the proper masculinity of Jesus was demonstrated insofar as his torturers did not "break him" allowing for him to signify the ultimate truth of his identity as the son of male/masculine deity and a human female.

But what of non-fiction narratives such as those developed by lawyers Deputy Assistant Attorney General John Yoo, Attorney General Alberto Gonzales, and Assistant Attorney General Jay S. Bybee; by politicians Secretary of Defense Donald Rumsfeld and President G.W. Bush; and by senior military persons General Geoffrey Miller and Lt. General Ricardo S. Sanchez, among others? Anthony Lewis wrote in the introduction to *The Torture Papers: The Road to Abu Ghraib* that the legal efforts "to argue away the rules against torture ... led to "mortal and political disaster" (in Greenberg and Dratel 2005, xiii) for the US, but even more so led to the institutionalization and legalization of cruel and inhumane engagement with other human beings, even if they are defined as the enemy. For example, Assistant Attorney General Jay S. Bybee advised Attorney General Alberto Gonzales that "[p]hysical pain amounting to torture must be equivalent in intensity to the pain accompanying serious physical injury such as organ failure impairment of bodily functions or even death" (ibid., xiii). Narrowly defining torture as organ failure, physical impairment and death meant that multiple forms of torture, varied and varying inscriptions of pain, and their deployment were on the table.

In legal discourses, documents were examined and interpreted by Yoo, Bybee, and others in such a way as to lay legal, and therefore rational, ground for the use of torture to ferret out the "truth" from the bodies of those humans marked as terrorists. First, the Iraqi men (and some women), often gathered up in military sweeps enacted in the streets of Abu Ghraib, Baghdad, and other cities throughout Iraq were not specified as enemy prisoners of war since they then would have come under the protection of the Third Geneva Convention:

> The then White House Counsel Alberto Gonzales [January 2002] opined that the war on terror had "render[ed] obsolete Geneva's strict limitations on questioning of enemy prisoners," and he recommend that the president deny al Qaeda and Taliban prisoners the protection of the Third Geneva Convention to "preserve flexibility" and "reduce the threat" that administration officials and military personnel would later be prosecuted for war crimes ... Stating that the war against terrorism had "usher[ed] in a new paradigm," President Bush formally endorsed this policy in a memorandum issued on February 7 [2002].
>
> (Jaffer and Singh 2007, 4)

Instead detainees were specified as al-Qaeda or Taliban terrorists (or potential terrorists) and "illegal combatants" and therefore "not entitled to Enemy Prisoner of War (EPW) status under the Geneva Conventions" (ibid., 7). Lewis wrote that much legal effort was given over to finding ways to define detainees as "unlawful combatants" that is non-state or failed state combatants (adopted by President Bush on January 9, 2002) in order to avoid charges of war crimes (in Greenberg and Dratel 2005, xiv) as well as mark those who would be tortured as liminal—outside of normative human social relations—and therefore the rules of warfare need not apply. However, it could not have been clear who was or was not a terrorist, and therefore a regime of pain, carefully and methodically applied, became a means to penetrate the Iraqi male (regardless of age) to reveal the "darkness" inside; a darkness that not only held the "truth" of his "terrorist" identity, but also the "truth" of his "kind" (non-white, Middle Eastern Islamic male/masculine).

To access the truth in the recesses of the Iraqi male body, John Yoo wrote a memorandum for the working group Donald Rumsfeld authorized in 2003 for the consideration of interrogation techniques. Yoo's infamous memorandum parroted Jay S. Bybee's:

> abuse does not rise to the level of torture under US law unless it inflicts pain "equivalent in intensity to the pain accompanying serious physical injury, such as organ failure, impairment of bodily function, or even death [quoting Yoo]." ... they [Yoo and Bybee] also argued that US laws banning torture could not constitutionally be applied to interrogations ordered by the president in his capacity as commander in chief of the armed forces, and that in any event,

the defenses of "necessary" and "self-defense" would "potentially eliminate criminal liability."

(Jaffer and Singh 2007, 14)

The ground was laid for the use of pain by legal counsel to the White House, and governmental officials (politicians really), Rumsfeld and Bush having secured legal justification of the internment and torture of "Middle Eastern terrorists" (aka Taliban and al-Qaeda) endorsed it arguing that under current circumstances, the so-called "new paradigm,"[14] the gloves must come off. Rumsfeld, putting General Michael E. Dunlavey in place to oversee interrogation at Guantánamo, indicated that "the Defense Department 'had accumulated a number of bad guys' and that 'he wanted a product and he wanted intelligence now'" (Jaffer and Singh 2007, 6). In a written directive of December 2, 2002, Rumsfeld authorized isolation for thirty days at a time, 24-hour interrogations, the use of guard dogs, and permission to:

> Deprive prisoners of light and auditory stimuli, forcibly strip them naked, hood them, and subject them to stress positions. Some of these methods were adapted from the SERE program, and many of them went far beyond the Army field Manual. Rumsfeld's directive plainly authorized interrogators to subject prisoners to "humiliating and degrading" treatment ...
>
> (Jaffer and Singh 2007, 8)

This directive was based on the 2002 government document entitled "JTF [Joint Task Force] GTMO [Guantánamo] SERE Interrogation SOP [Standard Operating Procedure]" (Jaffer and Singh 2007, 6)

Equally, the US military was involved in the use of pain to control and subjugate those persons marked as Middle Eastern terrorists. General Geoffrey Miller went to Abu Ghraib in August 2003 to assess interrogation methods. He felt that interrogators were hampered because they did not have complete control of prisoners' lives at all times. He therefore gave "military leaders in Iraq the list of interrogation methods that Rumsfeld had approved for use at Guantánamo" and recommending that "interrogators should make more aggressive use of military dogs" (ibid., 23–24). The attitudes of Rumsfeld and Miller opened the door for the wholesale implementation of the inscription of pain on the body of the detainees, even unto death, to acquire what was called "actionable intelligence" or intelligence that could be acted upon. Lt. General Ricardo S. Sanchez, at that time commander of coalition forces in Iraq, encouraged interrogators to:

> "go to the outer limits" to obtain information, and "Headquarters" pressed interrogators to "break" the prisoners. In August 2003, military interrogators

in Iraq were informed that the "gloves are coming off," that prisoners were to be "broken," and that the interrogators should propose "wish lists" of "effective" interrogation techniques for review.

(Jaffer and Singh 2007, 31)

Although there was some resistance from lawyers, politicians, and military personnel, deployed were discourses from the three sites of law, politics, and the military (among others such as the media) that rationalized and endorsed the use of torture to acquire the truth. But these discourses not only rationalized and endorsed torture, they assume without question that torture and truth were linked, a position similar to that of pre-eighteenth-century French legal courts. Indeed, Jaffer and colleagues noted that the FBI questioned the use of torture arguing that it was "ineffective and counterproductive" (Jaffer and Singh 2007, 17).[15]

Torture, Ritualized Pain, and the Male/Masculine Other: The Case of Abu Ghraib

If we begin with understanding, as Angela Carter (1990) did reading the Marquis de Sade, that the hand of whomever holds the whip is the hand of power and in a white, heterosexual, masculine hegemony it is a white masculine hand regardless of the gender of who holds it, we can account for white female/feminine US soldiers participating in the "softening up" and interrogation of the "security detainees" (also called unlawful combatants and terrorists) in the "hard site" of Abu Ghraib (Jaffer and Singh 2007, 33, 34). "Softening up" was the procedure that took place before, during, and after interrogation, and operated:

> on the basis of "pride up and ego down" and "futility"[16] ... [For example,] interrogators at Guantánamo stripped Mohammed al-Qahtani naked, subjected him to repeated strip searches, forced him to wear women's underwear on his head, led him around a room on a dog leash, and forced him to perform dog tricks. The perception [was] that such methods were authorized, [and were] combined with the understanding that military police were expected to "set the conditions" for fruitful interrogations ...

(Jaffer and Singh 2007, 26)

Some of this softening up of prisoners of war, along with the pain inflicted during interrogation led directly to the death of some of these men specified as Taliban or al-Qaeda and therefore Middle Eastern Islamic terrorists. These so-called terrorists were subjected to a multitude of bodily inscriptions wherein the indexical sign of pain was writ large within the parameters of torture.

Bound within the ritual of torture, there was a deflowering of the terrorist, a deflowering that made apparent not only the truth behind their lie that he was not a terrorist, but also the truth of his intrinsic femininity that would be forced from the recesses of his male body by the properly masculine hand of the torturer. The inscription of pain was ritually encapsulated and moved through three moments, as per Arnold van Gennep's model (1960): separation, or the removal of the detainee from their normative space in society to a space demarcated proper to the ritual: a liminal space wherein the terrorist-other was betwixt and between, called hard sites and where the normative rules of society did not apply. Here torture was viable and pain operated as the semiotic medium by which the rite of torture was given both its meaning and logic. The detainee, defined as terrorist or potential terrorist, and therefore an unlawful combatant, was equally made a liminal being in order to act as the fulcrum of the rite of torture. Upon completion of the rite, the newly inscribed detainee was returned to the prison population, to a hospital, or to death; and maybe even once and a while back home. Following van Gennep, each segment of the rite can also be a rite in itself, while all three segments (separation, liminality, and reintegration) come together to produce the entire rite: in this instance the rite of torture.

The spaces appointed to enclose torture were called "hard sites" or "black sites" and were shrouded in secrecy known only to the fully initiated: torturers and tortured. In this space prisoners, primarily male (of a variety of ages), were set apart from the rest of the prison population and designated as those who must participate in the rite of torture.[17] Here we see the first segment of the rite, as per Arnold van Gennep's theory of rites of passage, "initiates" ("ghost detainees" as they were called in Abu Ghraib), were set apart and "softened up" evidenced in the Abu Ghraib images leaked to the media in 2004. One "high-value" detainee reported to the International Committee of the Red Cross that he had been "hooded, handcuffed in the back, and made to lie face down, on a hot surface during transportation" which culminated in three months spent in hospital for burns (Greenberg and Dratel 2005, 390–391). Humiliation, shame, dismay, fear, despair and hopelessness were also aspects of this softening up and were evoked by the stripping "initiates" and forcing them to parade naked, sometimes in front of female interrogators, to wear women's undergarments on their heads or bodies, to publicly masturbate, to wear dog leashes; to pantomime (possibly perform) fellatio, and to do dog tricks. This was what the interrogators termed a variant of "pride and ego down" and was used to "'set the conditions' for fruitful interrogations ..." (Jaffer and Singh 2007, 27).

In association with the above, physical softening in this phase of the rite consisted of a number of the indexical signs of pain played out in: stress positions; environmental manipulation, such as extreme heat and cold, unending strobe lights and loud music; deprivation of sleep; constant physical training for hours; standing for long hours in one position;[18] hooding; and the use of dogs to intimidate or attack, among others (Jaffer and Singh 2007, 16–42). For example, Iraqi prisoners "would be taken to an empty swimming pool and handcuffed and leg-cuffed, hooded with burlap bags, and made to kneel for up to twenty-four hours awaiting interrogation" (ibid., 36).

The first phase of the rite of torture was composed of actions that would be frequently repeated when "initiates" were subjected to further torture in the interrogation room; the inner ritual space wherein the second phase, or liminality, of the rite of torture was enacted. In the interrogation space, a prescribed manner of torture was engaged. The "initiate" was fully introduced to the indexical sign of pain in the form of beatings with blunt force objects, often handcuffed in a stress position with hands behind the back to cell window bars. In some instances, as in the case of Abed Hamed Mowhoush, they died in this fashion. This was a failed torture session according to those who considered themselves to be technicians of torture (Rejali 2007, 450). Abed Hamed Mowhoush's autopsy report indicated that "this 56-year-old Iraqi detainee died of asphyxiation due to smothering and chest compression. Significant findings of the autopsy included rib fractures and numerous contusions (bruises), some of which were patterned due to impacts with a blunt object(s) ..." (Jaffer and Singh 2007, 27). Included with the pain of bruised and battered flesh was a dousing with cold water and then a subjection to cold temperatures and/or the infamous water boarding. The kinds of torture vary, but the inscription of the indexical sign of pain on all aspects of the flesh including cognition to access the "truth" was a constant. Interrogation went on for hours, in some instances was twenty hours out of every twenty-four for days in a row (ibid., 7).

The interrogations of the second phase of the rite of torture were a relentless and insistent movement toward a third and final phase, incorporation, wherein the initiate takes on the identity proffered to them: in this instance the subjugated Middle Eastern Islamic male or the feminized other of the orientalist fantasy (Stoler 2002). In this rite of torture, the etching of pain was seen to have torn away all edifices of identity to reveal an innate femininity; femininity demonstrated by the tumbling words given over in desperation, the cries, screams, the begging, or in death when they succumbed to torturer-priests who governed the space, the body, and the indexical sign of pain. Death was also a revelation of intrinsic femininity, and therefore otherness, as evidenced by the images of an Iraq male who died during an interrogation (November 24, 2003) by "other governmental agencies" (OGA, but thought to be almost exclusively as CIA). His body was placed in the shower area of the hard site within Abu Ghraib whereupon the body bag was opened so that CPL Charles Graner and SPC Sabrina Harman could ghoulishly take pictures of the dead man. In one picture SPC Harman is shown leaning over the dead man making a thumbs up gesture while smiling into the camera held by CPL Graner (Scherer and Benjamin 2006). Clearly this image speaks of domination and power in the hands of those, Graner and Harman, who were seen clowning with the dead body. As Bruce Lincoln has written:

> It is their intent to demonstrate dramatically and in public the *powerlessness* of the image and thereby to inflict a double disgrace on its champions, first by exposing the bankruptcy of their vaulted symbols and, second, their impotence in the face of attack.
>
> (Lincoln 1989, 120)

Those who succumbed to pain, either through speaking the "truth" or dying were gathered up under the sign of feminized other, which signified a subjugated and powerless Middle Eastern Islamic masculinity—even if that speaking was a fiction (much as President Bush's 2003 "Mission Accomplished" photo opportunity was a fiction).

The third phase, operating within van Gennep's model, brings the ritual to a close with the incorporation of so-called Middle Eastern Islamic terrorists under the sign of an abject and defeated "masculine" other. A boundary between masculinities was drawn, and each act of interrogation redrew that boundary in the flesh of the "other" in the application of the indexical sign of pain. Pain also acted to signify a boundary between those who suffered the pain and those who applied the pain, but even as the boundary was written in the flesh it was breached as the torturer and tortured are intimately bound brought together as they are in the rite of torture. And, because the boundary between the torturer and tortured is but a fiction, it must be redrawn again and again to give it the credence of materiality through constant repetition.

The administers of pain, the interrogators, belonged to a secret club, one more than likely defined in relation to masculinity (regardless that those marked as female participate), whose comings and goings were clandestine and whose power was unknown, as it was unclear to whom they were accountable. They oversaw the black and hard sites, and those outside of the interrogation rooms directed to "soften up" detainees, such as Lynndie England, Sabrina Harman, and George Graner (among others), were their willing assistants who mimed their superiors hoping for power and approval. The women moved between roles of donning US white masculinity and standing on the sidelines properly feminine, admiring and supporting it (Enloe 2004, 99–118): as in any normative pecking order where the "strong"—warrior-soldier—are understood to dominant the "weak." In the rite of torture, the "strong" are established through the inscription of the indexical sign of pain onto the body of the other, while the "weak" are established as other through the unwilling reception of, and response to, pain. In the rite of torture, pain signified power and powerlessness. It was also used within the paradigm of the rite of torture to signify those willing to administer pain as bravely engaging with "darkness" in order to overcome "evil." Overcoming this so-called evil (the terrorist) allowed white US masculine power to reassert its domination both locally and globally. Breaking the bodies of those who dared to penetrate them leaving a gaping hole in the New York skyline required, the US argued, the use of torture.

Concluding Comments: Pain and the Colonized Body— Microcosm and Macrocosm

> Religion in its entirety was founded upon sacrifice. But only an interminable detour allows us to reach that instant where the contraries seem visibly joined, where religious horror disclosed in sacrifice becomes linked to the abyss of eroticism, to the last shuddering tears that eroticism alone can illuminate (Bataille 1989, 207).

In many ways ritualized torture speaks of a return of the repressed; the repressed as erotic desire expressed through the indexical sign of pain encapsulated and justified in ritual. Inquisitors of the medieval and early modern periods of the Catholic Church worked with other governmental, ecclesiastical, and medical officials to pry open and expose false belief in the bodies of those considered heretics, and later, witches and sorcerers. The inquisitors were the authoritative knowers who determined those who would be subjected to the rite of torture.

The ritual use of pain, indeed the use of ritual itself, however, is an anathema to Protestantism. Ritual spectacle is an "idolatry" of the Catholic Church (and Orthodox Christian Churches), an idolatry rejected in the past and a current reminder of the boundary between Catholics and Protestants. Protestants, in general, understand themselves as their own masters since the Bible acts as a source of authority rather than a hierarchy of priests wielding ritual. Ritual spectacle, pomp and ceremony, relics, icons, and miracles were left behind as Protestant groups began to define themselves in the United States. Why then would ritual spectacle, spectacle insofar as operating as a public secret, rear its head in an institution that represented itself in generic Protestant terms? Could it be that dominant, white, and heterosexual US masculinity was at risk in the current global climate? Could it be that the masculinity of United States as a player on the militarized global stage was feminized, and therefore destabilized, when the towers were penetrated? Or could it be that since the attack was seen to have been perpetrated by those occupying the "third worlds"; the racialized "lesser," they should be made to suffer to atone for their sin?

The "hows," however, can be as interesting as the "whys." I am interested in how ritual and pain were (and continue to be) brought together and etched on the body to signify the errancy of those marked as other. In the ritual of torture pain is the mirror by which the feminine was exposed in the bodies of the penetrated other, while absence of pain of the unpenetrated torturer signified the return of proper US masculinity on the global stage. When the twin towers were penetrated, this penetration signified the vulnerability of white, US, Protestant, capitalism (they were the trade towers after all). Furthermore, as towers that marked US military and economic hegemony, they also signified as the twin phalli, both declined, of course, in the masculine. From this event arose the effort to reassert and emphatically pronounce US masculine hegemonic power. This assertion came in the form of war while its emphatic pronouncement came in the form of standing above the law, all law. The ritual use of pain, then, became a means by which to demonstrate the authority to define the so-called "war on terror"; a way to make apparent one's position above International law (when all others are held accountable to it); and ultimately the rightness and righteousness of one's position. And since one's position is right and proper so too must be the masculinity of the nation. The penetration of the marked body (brown, Islamic, non-western, non-Anglo, etc.) through torture allowed for the reclamation and reassertion of the masculinity that was put at risk by the attack on the twin towers on that day in 2001.

Equally, as suggested above, there was a metaphysical play since deity was regularly brought into the picture by all the players in the game of military dominance. In the so-called "war against terror" fought on the soil of Iraq and Afghanistan, the generally Protestant Christian deity of the US and the Islamic deity of the Middle East were sign-symbols made to speak the power, truth, and righteousness of national boundaries and masculine identities. In the struggle to locate and fix those who were "evil doers" and those who fought them, the ritualized use of the indexical sign of pain allowed representatives of the United States to inscribe the mark of evil onto the fleshy bodies of the other, much as the word "rapist" was written on the body of one of the detainees, exposing the "real', that is the truth, hidden in the recesses of the body—they are weak and feminine succumbing to the indexical sign of pain. Furthermore, by inscribing the emasculated flesh of the other as the site of evil (and through them their deity) the uninscribed masculine flesh of the "same" (white, US, and seemingly heterosexual masculine) stands as the site of good (and through them their deity). US masculine domination of the globe is once again proclaimed to be true through the inscription of the indexical sign of pain onto the bodies of the emasculated other.

Chapter 5

Cut to the Bone
Pain, Foreskins, and Masculinities

> [G]enealogy retrieves an indispensable restraint: it must record the singularity of events outside of any monotonous finality; it must seek them in the most unpromising places, in what we tend to feel is without history-in sentiments, love, conscience, instincts; it must be sensitive to their recurrence, not in order to trace the gradual curve of their evolution, but to isolate the different scenes where they engaged in different roles. Finally, genealogy must define even those in stances when they are absent, the moment when they remained unrealized (Plato, at Syracuse, did not become Mohammed).
> (Foucault 1984, 76)

Introduction

The foreskin of the penis has been, and continues to be, of significant importance for many social groups, not the least of which for the Eurowest and its mainstream dominant systems of belief and practice Christianities (and Judaisms and Islams). The kind of importance linked to the foreskin depends on the context and perceived outcomes associated with its presence, absence, and excision. In some contexts it is a feminine veil (Silverman 2004) that must be removed in order to secure the full potential of masculinity, in others it is a site of impurity that must be cut away to protect the penis, the body (Kacker et al. 2012), and even the soul (Scolnic 2013), while in other contexts its cutting away was and is the only means to embody purity and to achieve identity (Zucconi 2007; Boyarin 1992).

Keeping the foreskin and penis in mind in the analysis of male circumcision and pain, the focus of this chapter ensures that the body and the body in pain remain in view regardless that the bodies represented in my text are, and have already been, abstracted through textualization.[1] *Circumcision* is a process, whether a medical procedure, a rite, or a strategy, that produces a result; the removal of the foreskin from the head of a penis. The three bodily outcomes of circumcision—the penis without a fleshy covering, the discarded foreskin, and the pain—are overdetermined, carrying so much weight as to run aground on any one of the determinants that accompany these sign-symbols of masculinities. Interwoven with other sign-symbols such as the phallus (which is never veiled, covered, or enfleshed), the foreskin is that which is discarded and seen as other/impure, often associated with the feminine and/or the abject (Kristeva 1987); the defleshed penis signifies as a pure, proper, and healthy masculinity. The pain of the cut can be heroically engaged (potential warriors), erased (infants), or ignored (patients). The outcomes of male circumcision, that is the cut, the discarded foreskin and the pain, indexically mark the bodies of babies, children, youth, and adults acting as a dense transfer point of power (Foucault 1978). Here is a site where masculine power is ritually recalled, recognized, and transferred, while those on whom this pain, mixed with pleasure, is conferred are recognized as potentially proper (or improper when uncircumcised) masculine males.

The penis is at the center of the ideology of the normative interconnection of penis, phallus, and masculine power. Kaja Silverman (1992, 15–51) discusses this intersection, writing that it is the penis/phallus formation that operates as the dominate fiction of masculine hegemonies and indeed in such hegemonic relations if there is an interruption of the alignment of the penis and phallus, then reality itself is called into question, "the entire 'world' ... depends upon the alignment of phallus and penis" (ibid., 16). And this alignment is neither natural nor normative, but must be achieved, and one method is ritual circumcision, wherein the offending abjection—the foreskin—is removed. This removal brings into existence the alignment of which the result is the proper male/masculine, however that is defined within particular social and historical locations wherein the event of circumcision is deployed.

This chapter investigates circumcision as it has been represented in modern and ancient texts in order to ask how pain in the representation of circumcision signifies: I ask how the cut, the foreskin, and the pain associated with it are central to the construction of masculinities, locating masculinities, along with the foreskin, penis, and phallus, in human ontology (penis) and metaphysics (phallus), both of which reify and mystify masculinities, the penis, and circumcision. It is my view that the cut that runs deep, the discarded foreskin and the pain that links them are indexical signs that naturalize the penis/phallus alignment, the latter of which acts to root and enhance mythemes of masculinity. To do this work I draw on five textualized moments/events, ancient and modern, to construct a loose genealogy of circumcision, beginning in the current period and ending in ancient Egypt, where can be found some of the earliest images of this ancient rite that continues to shape representations of the male/masculine. Tracking these moments reveals the construction of masculinity through circumcision and the passage of pain that accompanies the cut. As indexical signs, pain and the cut bring into existence a gendered identity rooted in the penis as "manflesh" and the phallus as "manspirit."

Penile Contentions: The Foreskin as Ugly, Beautiful, Fetid, and Fragrant

Before engaging the event of circumcision, one might consider what circumcision removes and how that slip of flesh is perceived. The foreskin is a loose piece of flesh, the prepuce, that covers the head of the penis. Nicola Zampieri, Emanuela Pianezzola, and Cecilia Zampieri (2008, 1305) note that: "It is now known that the foreskin, or prepuce is the principal location of erogenous sensation in human males, and removal of the prepuce substantially reduces such sensations." To their minds efforts to reduce sexual pleasure can, and often do, represent an understanding of sexuality as problematic. For some a penis left in a natural state (i.e., without the removal of the foreskin) was seen as impure, and leading to sexual licentiousness and sexually transmitted diseases. The loose flesh of the foreskin was abject, a thing of filth. Connected to a state of impurity, the foreskin was removed by ancient Egyptian priests (Zucconi 2007), observant Jews (Scolnic 2013) and Moroccan Muslims. In US mid- to late-nineteenth-century medical views, circumcision was proposed as curative for a number of medical conditions. As Adam Henerey wrote:

> Around this time, physicians were starting to develop therapeutic connections to circumcision within their practices. One of the most notable examples was the career of Lewis Sayre. In his years as a physician and surgeon, he found in cases of orthopedic dysfunction, hernia, dyspepsia, epilepsy, and even paralysis that circumcision caused varying forms of improvement.
> (Henerey 2004, 269)

Others believe that the penis with an attached foreskin meant increased sexual deviance and therefore circumcision was employed to prevent masturbation, a practice thought to bring about decrepitude in the male/masculine. Progress, the progress of society and the progress of "man," informed most nineteenth-century theories of the human species. Progress and social evolutionism were linked, and "man's" progress could be halted by his own lack of control: the lack of which could be seen in the fate of the poor, the lower classes, the subjugated peoples under colonialist empires, and, as always, the hysterical woman. The individual who leads a licentious life, the physician and university professor John Cowan wrote in 1897 in his *Science of a New Life*, "causes a great drain on his vitality—such a drain as required the whole life force of his system to supply" (Cowan, 1970, 120). Consequently, a sexually "spendthrift" man (and in this equation onanistic boys) "does in part or in whole, weaken his nervous system ... and dyspepsia, rheumatism, apoplexy, paralysis and a score of other diseases, assert their sway" (ibid., 118).

In rites of circumcision the foreskin can be taken to be a "feminine veil" that must be removed in order that the boy become a proper man (Delaney 1995, 60; Juschka 2020). Linked to circumcision the foreskin signifies as abject and a threat to the physical, mental, sexual, and spiritual health of humans marked as male/masculine. The foreskin with its sensitivity meant the penis was even more susceptible to the sexual instinct and subsequently the male/masculine might devolve becoming less civilized and more susceptible to things like aggressive or so-called deviant sexuality, superstition, gambling, sexually transmitted illness such as syphilis, alcoholism and/or any other psycho-physio illness that hinged on the presence and absence of the foreskin.[2] One doctor noted that "life-insurance companies should class the wearer of the prepuce under the head of hazardous risks" (Gollaher 2000, 14).

This understanding of the foreskin as something polluting and excessively sexual haunts the current efforts of medicine to stay the course of HIV/AIDs in countries across the African continent. The World Health Organization takes the position that circumcision is a preventative surgery for HIV/AIDS. According to the WHO, fifteen million males in fourteen African countries have been circumcised as a means to prevent the transmission of HIV (World Health Organization 2017). As abject, the foreskin is imbued with the power of otherness that is a threat and, therefore, must be contained.

The power of otherness situates the foreskin in the same liminal space that is shared by deities and other beings allowing the foreskin, then, to participate in the magical and mystical, palpitating with power. Maurice Bloch wrote in his study of the Merina in Madagascar that a senior relative ate the foreskin immediately after it was removed from the child's penis (1986, 79). In this context the foreskin was associated with blessings and fertility, while in different contexts other kinds of power are associated with the foreskin. The foreskin of the figure of Jesus in Christian mythology, for example, was a relic of the medieval world, said to have been given to Charlemagne by an angelic visitor. Charlemagne turned the relic over to the Church where it was housed in the pope's private collection until it was stolen in 1527 during the destruction of Rome. However, it was recovered and the elite women of Rome were able to enjoy its "sublime odor" as they described its smell (Gollaher 2000), while St. Bridget (Birgitta) of fourteenth-century Sweden swooned at the taste of Jesus's foreskin (Shell 1997, 346–347). Connected to a deity the foreskin signified as divine and otherworldly and, according to ancient Christian polemicists such as the venerated John Chrysostom (fourth century CE) and

Severus of Antioch (fifth to sixth centuries CE) would be rejoined to the penis of Jesus when the end of times arrived (Jacobs 2012, 91). It seems in Christian thought the mark taken to represent Jewish identity must be removed from the body of its deity.

Text One—HIV/AIDS, Africa, and the Black Penis: Circumcision and Control

In the twenty-first century the foreskin continues to signify beyond its fleshing presence. Like the clitoris, the penis is hooded, and it is the hood that has and continues to draw attention. The attention it receives is critical insofar as the hood is taken to be a vector, or at least a potential vector, of disease, dirt, and impurities. Infant, youth and adult male circumcision have been employed as a means to prevent disease, the more recent being the transmission of HIV wherein the foreskin is seen to amass disease. David Cooper and colleagues approvingly cite the World Health Organization in their article supporting infant circumcision as a method to reduce and eradicate HIV infections in Australia:

> The World Health Organization, the Joint United Nations Programme on HIV/AIDS and the Global Fund to Fight AIDS, Tuberculosis and Malaria have endorsed male circumcision to control HIV attributed to heterosexual contact in hyperendemic areas, stating: "The efficacy of male circumcision in reducing female to male transmission of HIV has been proven beyond reasonable doubt. This is an important landmark in the history of HIV prevention."
> (Cooper et al. 2010, 218)

The "proven" however, is based on the three African trials that have been questioned because of problems in the study. Robert Darby and Robert Van Howe wrote that:

> Perhaps the most crucial flaw in these three studies is that the researchers assumed that all the men who became HIV positive during the course of the trials were infected through sexual contact. When the study results are examined closely, there is evidence that as many as half the infections could have been acquired non-sexually.
> (Darby and Van Howe 2011, 460)

Darby and Van Howe further show, drawing on the work of A. Garenne (2008), that there was no significant difference between circumcised and uncircumcised men in eight African countries when it came to the presence of the HIV seroprevalence; that in three African countries circumcised men showed a higher prevalence; and that it is only in two African countries that uncircumcised men showed a higher prevalence of HIV. Furthermore, they write, "in South Africa a third of the population is circumcised [and] HIV prevalence is among the highest on record" (Darby and Van Howe 2011, 460).

In the decision to circumcise males in Africa, the unequal global relations of countries were not taken into account, nor were the histories of colonization and the enslavement of black Africans by white Europeans. Relations of racist and economic domination shaped all interaction leading to some of the most horrific and genocidal actions by Eurowesterners and some of the most unbearable suffering endured by peoples of the African continent. Adam Hochschild's study of the appalling conditions of colonialism in the Congo Free State under the so-called philanthropic actions of King Leopold exposes the greed, terror and murderous sadism that fueled the collection of rubber for white peoples' cars, bicycle tires, and other commodities. As Hochschild shows, quoting Charles Lemaire Belgium's first commission of the equator district (1890–1894), "to gather rubber ... one must cut off hands, noses and ears" (Hochschild 1998, 165). The scale of torture and murder of the people of central Africa is a horror buried in the depths of time, but one that presaged the mutilation, torture, and murder that would be enacted against the people of Sierra Leone in the 1990s during the procurement of diamonds, called blood diamonds. Greg Campbell wrote:

> But their signature war crime was amputation. In response to Sierra Leone president Ahmad Tejan Kabbah's 1996 plea for his countrymen to "join hands" for peace, the RUF [Revolutionary United Front] began dismembering their victims and dumping the body parts on the steps of the presidential palace. Although hands were the most common limb severed, the RUF also sliced off civilians' lips, ears, legs, breasts, and tongues to inspire terror.
>
> (Campbell 2012)

A history of slavery, mutilation, and the slaughter of millions, and yet the World Health Organization considered it "voluntary"—how can it be voluntary when people are told that male circumcision prevents the spread of HIV even if, as Darby and Howe note heterosexual sexual contact is not the only means the disease is spreading. How racism and colonialism shape the conceptualization and practice of circumcision should have been the first step in the research of male circumcision. If they had done this the WHO would have been aware of circumcision's uses and abuses throughout history. As David Gollaher has written concerning circumcision in the mid-twentieth-century United States:

> That no scientific research validated the theory that circumcision inhibited the spread of venereal disease did not keep physicians from continuing to promote the view that it did. In the wake of World War II, for example, *Newsweek* magazine quoted Dr. Eugene Hand's address to the AMA in which he observed that whereas the "promiscuous" and uncircumcised Negro had an incidence of venereal infection of "almost 100% ... for the widely educated Jew, circumcised at birth, the venereal disease rate has remained the same or decreased."
> (Gollaher 2000, 25)

Male circumcision as a preventative to acquiring HIV continues to be the view of the WHO and the majority of the medical community, but the application of this knowledge is limited to countries of Africa as voluntary medical male circumcision is not engaged in Eurowestern countries such as United States and Canada, even though both countries continue to show increased numbers of HIV infections. In Canada there were 2,402 new diagnoses in 2017, an increase of 17.1% since 2014. However, treatment is not circumcision; rather education, testing and drug treatment are the methods for dealing with the continued HIV epidemic in Canada (Haddad et al. 2018, 324). The US reported 38,739 new cases of HIV in 2017 (Centers for Disease Control and Prevention 2018, 22) and the majority are male. There have not, however, been efforts to institute voluntary male circumcision in the US. Certainly the number of new HIV infections in Africa are much higher than the US and Canada, but South Africa, a target for voluntary male circumcision, continues to experience high numbers of new infections, and according to a 2012 survey "The incidence analysis suggests that there is no evidence that incidence among adults aged 15–49 years has changed between 2008 and 2012" (Shisana et al. 2014, 113). The age bracket are those males primarily targeted for circumcision suggest that male circumcision is less efficacious than suggested and it is certainly not the magic bullet for the prevention of HIV transmission. As Olive Shisana and colleagues suggest, education about HIV/AIDs is key as South Africans remain at risk due to misinformation about the transmission of HIV leading to people believing they are not at risk (ibid., 114; see also Rehle et al. 2015). As in the past, colonial powers, now under the rubric of development and aid, consistently find the African male body to be problematic and in need of adjustment and alteration. The epidemic of HIV/AIDs is spread throughout the globe, but it is the African penis, particularly the black African penis, that comes under censure.

In the many discussions concerning voluntary male circumcision there is no reference to the pain of circumcision. Cutting the foreskin from the head of a penis is not painless; it is full of pain. Why is there a lack of register of pain? What might this lack tell us about white Eurowestern attitudes toward the racialized male African body and his penis? As Hochschild has shown in his study of the Belgian Congo, among most whites the African was more animal than human, and therefore did not feel pain like a proper (that is, white, Eurowestern) human:

> What made it possible for the functionaries in the Congo to so blithely watch the *chicotte*[3] in action and, as we shall see, to deal out pain and death in other ways as well? To begin with, of course, was race. To Europeans, Africans were inferior beings: lazy, uncivilized; little better than animals. In fact, the most common way they were put to work was, like animals, as beasts of burden. In any system of terror, the functionaries must first of all see the victims as less than human, and Victorian ideas about race provided such a foundation.
> (Hochschild 1998, 121)

Marked as more animal than human meant the pain, anguish, and loss of Indigenous peoples in the Belgian Congo could no more signify than the pain of a calf slaughtered in front of its mother or a horse beaten to death in the streets. It was common practice in the eighteenth-century Eurowest to torture non-human animals for entertainment with dogs whipped and killed on St. Luke's Day, and "untold numbers of cats tortured on all days—tied up in bags, hung from May poles, suspended from ropes, burned at the stake, chased flaming through the streets and incinerated by the sack load" (Kalof 2007, 112). In England the nineteenth century saw vivisection of live animals for so-called medical science and although women organized against vivisection, they did not carry the day: elite, white, men—medical students—ensured the practice continued (ibid., 140), even until today when millions of non-human animals continue to die in science experiments. For many of the Enlightenment, in line with René Descartes's view, non-human animals do not feel pain and any crying, screaming, or distress is purely instinctual. This is the kind of logic that shaped colonialism and the interaction between the oppressive and dominant Eurowest and the African peoples it sought to enslave and/or slaughter. The cutting off of the foreskin of millions of male Africans without recognition of the pain of the act or the implications in light of the colonial past signify, once again, how Eurowestern powers continue to enact white racism and colonialism against African black bodies.[4]

Text Two—Infant Circumcision and the Erasure of Pain

If circumcision was "voluntary" for the almost fifteen million black males of the countries of Africa, this is certainly not the case for male infants who were regularly circumcised in many Eurowestern locations in the nineteenth and twentieth centuries. Male infant circumcision was engaged as a means to prevent and cure sexually transmitted infections, for illnesses of the body and mind, and to quell the madness of masturbation. Adam Henerey notes that surgeons such as Lewis Sayre used circumcision to correct or improve "orthopedic dysfunction, hernia, dyspepsia, epilepsy and even paralysis" (Henerey 2004, 269). Male circumcision was the one-stop fix for many disorders, particularly sexual disorders such as sexual aggression and "masturbatory insanity" (ibid.). Further to this moral medicalization, by the early twentieth century circumcision begins to signify in terms of class and a physician/hospital birth of the middle class over and against a midwife/home birth of the working class. Developed in line with middle- and upper-class moralism, the uncircumcised penis signified as "dirty" just as the lower classes were considered the "unwashed." It is at this time that male infant circumcision became a normative medical procedure (ibid., 270) enacted on the bodies of male infants.

Male infant circumcision had been supported by the medical community in the US, Canada, and the UK until its taken-for-granted use, like tonsillectomies, was challenged. With this challenge the 1960s and 1970s saw pediatric associations in these countries reverse their position, now stating that there were no medical reasons to routinely circumcise infants since the benefits were minor to nonexistent (Dave et al. 2003; Henerey 2004, 270–271; Sorokan, Finlay, and Jefferies 2015, 311). Neonatal circumcision began to fall off in all three countries, while the surgery continued to be more strongly supported in the US with the American Academy of Pediatrics again approving of the surgery when parents desired it and supported third-party payers for the surgery (Blank et al. 2012, 756). In instances of support of circumcision, such as by the American Academy of Pediatrics, the control and containment of STIs and HIV are cited as the primary reason to practice infant male circumcision (ibid., 756), regardless that there is no of evidence of such. S. S. Dave and colleagues (2003, 500) comment:

> [We] did not find any significant differences in the proportion of circumcised and uncircumcised British men reporting ever being diagnosed with any STI (11.1% compared with 10.8%, p = 0.815), bacterial STIs (6.4% cf 5.9%, p = 0.628), or viral STIs (4.7% cf 4.5%, p = 0.786) (table 1). We also found no significant associations between circumcision and being diagnosed with any one of the seven specific STIs.
>
> (Dave et al. 2003, 500)

Furthermore, even as the number of males circumcised is greater in the US than Canada and the UK, so too the number of HIV/AIDs infections. As Darby and Van Howe write:

> Both the United States and Indonesia, with predominantly circumcised male populations, have a significantly higher incidence of HIV than Australia, Canada, Britain and New Zealand, where circumcision is in decline or extremely rare. In the United States, African-Americans exhibit both the highest rate of circumcision and the highest rate of heterosexually-transmitted HIV.
>
> (Darby and Van Howe 2011, 460)

The debate continues about the value and ethical motives of infant male circumcision. Infants are not in the position to consent to the surgery and so their parents provide proxy consent, a dubious consent, argues Robert Van Howe as proxy consent should only be enacted in cases of medical necessity, something infant male circumcision is decidedly not (Van Howe 2013, 30). Van Howe further comments that when reaching the age of consent males in the US can then have themselves circumcised if they so desire. Eldar Sarajlic and Robert Darby further raise the "open future argument" wherein children have "rights in trust"; that is, rights they can take up when they reach adulthood. In light of these rights, the open future argument suggests that infant circumcision, even if it does no harm, violates the child's right to an open future by closing off some options for him in adulthood" (Sarajlic 2014, 337; Darby 2013).

The tendency of those who are proponents of infant male circumcision as a means to prevent STIs and HIV/AIDS is to consider larger social concerns over and against the concerns of the targeted group and the individuals of the group—a practice that raises some ethical concerns particularly in light of past practice. For example, the Tuskegee study of Untreated Syphilis in the African Americans in the US from the 1930 until the early 1970s where the control group remained infected and untreated, and a two year study to determine the health benefits of a children's diet using Indigenous children in residential schools wherein some were provided nutritious food while the control group was not (Juschka 2017). As with the Tuskegee study, further illnesses and death of the control group resulted. Both studies were directed toward the betterment of the larger social body at the cost of racialized and oppressed "other."

Those who support infant circumcision do not engage the pain of circumcision in any significant way, nor do they consider the possibility of trauma. The American Academy of Pediatrics comments that "nonpharmacologic techniques:" such as "positioning" or "sucrose pacifiers" are insufficient to control the pain the infant endures, and recommend the use of analgesia (Blank et al. 2012, 757). There appears to be a dismissal of infant pain, or at least the idea that there is significant pain and in earlier days pain intervention was non-existent or minimal, as the above quote suggests insofar as the infant was given a sugared soother. The idea that infants do not feel the pain of circumcision is an old one (Van Howe and Svoboda 2008) and reflects a belief similar to that held regarding the bodies of black Africans and their lack of refined nerves—the two beliefs connect in relation to a distorted evolutionary theory that locates the not fully formed or the racialized human as closer to nature and all that resides in nature are objects rather than subjects in this kind of ontology. Located in nature, male black African and infant bodies are conceptually located closer to non-human animals, who according to human hubris don't feel pain or feel it less significantly: apparently the fewer rights, the less pain experienced. Furthermore, in the work of proponents of infant male circumcision, the pain and shock of circumcision are never engaged as potentially traumatic or a trauma that marks one's life. However, there are men who have lamented their lost foreskin and have been haunted by the pain and shock (Boyle et al. 2002). Robert Darby and Laurence Cox's study of men circumcised as infants or young children write of the fear, loss, and distrust of humans that resulted from the circumcision event. As one Australian participant wrote: "I can't talk about the emotional side of how I feel affected by my circumcision. It's like a block, a secret—an atrocity. I've lost the right to self-direction and decision" (Darby and Cox 2008, 163). Rather than submit his infant son to this procedure, Michael Kimmel reflects on his choice not to circumcise his son in "The Kindest Un-cut: Feminism, Judaism and My Son's Foreskin." He wrote: "We had decided not to circumcise our son. Although he enters a world filled with violence, he would enter it without violence done to him. Although he will no doubt suffer many cuts and scrapes during his life, he would not bleed by our hand" (Kimmel 2001, 43).

Text Three—Circumcision and Pain in the Pauline, Philoic, and Josephean Texts

The Pauline letters are the primary site for the construction of a heroic figure central to Christian mythologies be they Catholic, Orthodox, or Protestant. In Catholic and Orthodox Christianities the letters are the divinely inspired works of a saint and apostle, while in Protestantisms these letters were, and remain, foundational to the construction of their systems of belief and practice (Seesengood 2010, 148–164). The letters number thirteen, although it is largely agreed only seven are authentically Pauline, while six are considered pseudepigraphical, written by those who wished to draw on the authority of the figure of Paul.

The figure of Paul is also presented in the text "Acts of the Apostles" where he is presented as a heroic figure, "a churchly actor, hero, martyr," suggests William Arnal (2011, 206), one who emulates the trials and tribulations of the deity he is represented as having espoused. The text of Acts is a myth of place and peoples, and in it two separate streams of followers, Jewish and Gentile, are woven together.[5] In this mythic narrative the figure of Paul was linked to the Gentiles and to the letters themselves attributed to, as they are, an author named Paul.[6]

The Pauline letters engage many subjects and circumcision is one that comes up repeatedly as a sticking point, a sticking point of what it meant to follow the deity proposed in the letters. The deity in the Pauline letters, Jesus Christ, is linked to another deity, the deity of the Jews called *Kyrios* or *Theos*[7] in the letters, a deity understood to have a significant and singular relationship with the Jews. However, this exclusive deity of the Jews could be extended to non-Jews through the semi-divine son. According to the Pauline letters, then, the path to salvation came in two forms: adherence to the law, and in this to the rite of circumcision, or through a new proposition, baptism—real and metaphoric—in the holy spirit (Romans 9–11; see also Thiessen 2011, 148; Livesey 2007, 144–152). Furthermore, the sense is not one pathway succeeding the other; rather, there are two pathways with one for the Jews, which included infant circumcision, and one for the Gentiles, which excluded circumcision and instead embraced baptism. For Gentiles the rite of circumcision was replaced by the rite of baptism since they were not Jews and therefore did not follow the law.

Condemning the need for circumcision of non-Jews, the Philippians' letter speaks of Paul having been circumcised on the eighth day and belonging to the "people of Israel, of the tribe of Benjamin, a Hebrew born of Hebrews; as to the law a Pharisee ..." (3:5). Set first in the list of identity markers, circumcision is the cut that allowed the formation of the identity that flowed from the rite (Arnal 2008, 75 ff.). The protagonist in the letter, Paul, is a Jew precisely because he followed a path that began with circumcision and led to adherence to, and support of, the law.

Being a law-abiding Jew, however, did not preclude interaction with deity, as the letter of Philippians insists locating its protagonist, Paul, in both arenas of circumcision and baptism. Locating Paul in both arenas constructs him as a liminal or interstitial figure and therefore a very useful apostle: He knows the law as a "Pharisee" and the spirit "because Christ Jesus has made [him] his own" (Phil. 2:12). Sharing in both, the protagonist Paul is authoritative in a way those who act in one or the other arena cannot be since the protagonist Paul, circumcised and baptized, can serve both the father and the son and therefore represents an ideal messenger. Certainly the other apostles are located as Jews in the New Testament texts, but their circumcisions are never referenced nor attested to: indeed, circumcision does not figure at all. It is in the letters of Paul that circumcision acts to signify identity and establish kinds: the circumcised Jew from the uncircumcised Gentile, but both baptized. Both rites proffer an identity to go with the rites; followers of the law and word, and followers of the word.

At no point in the Pauline letters does the discussion of the pain of circumcision surface, regardless that such pain might have operated as a convincing deterrent to adult circumcision, something the letters' protagonist is interested in doing. This absence of reference to the pain of circumcision could register a lack of consideration for the pain of infants, or for pain in general,[8] but it also may suggest that pain is not a deterrent and indeed to be properly masculine one did not flinch from it—a not uncommon view in the ancient Roman world within which the letters were shaped. Even the crucifixion of the partially divine Jesus, the ghost of whom appears to haunt the protagonist of the letters, did not stir the embers of pity for the pain endured by this half-deity: pain is elided and instead the texts propose the idea of the suffering of the deity in the form of suffering of the heart, mind and soul, but not flesh. Furthermore, such suffering was to be embraced by those who would follow the path of this deity. For example, Phil. 1:29, "For unto you it is given in the behalf of Christ, not only to believe on him, but also to suffer for his sake"; and Romans 8:17, "heirs of God, and joint-heirs with Christ; if so be that we suffer with him, that we may be also glorified together." The protagonist, Paul, must suffer in order to serve the deity, just as Moses and Jesus had suffered. Suffering is accorded value in the texts, but not bodily pain, which is absent. Although the indexical sign of pain appears absent, it is recalled by the trace of the cut circling the penis, signifying identity and commitment to the deity within the law, giving it presence in the Pauline letters.

Philo and Josephus both lived in and around the time of the Pauline letters. Works attributed to Philo are dated to his life span, circa 20 BCE to 40 CE. The texts of Philo, like the Pauline letters, discuss the subject of circumcision, but unlike Paul Philo commented on the pain of circumcision:

> [S]o as without examination to condemn the folly of mighty nations [Egypt in this instance], recollecting that it is not probable that so many myriads should be circumcised in every generation, mutilating the bodies of themselves and their nearest relations, in a manner which is accompanied with severe pain, without adequate cause.
>
> (Philo 1993b, SL I: 3)

Having raised pain, the author then sets alongside the pain of circumcision the pain of disease writing that circumcision is:

> a preventive for a painful disease, and of an affliction difficult to be cured, which they call a carbuncle ... Secondly it secures the cleanliness of the whole body in a way that is suited to the people consecrated to God ... Thirdly, there is the resemblance of the part that is circumcised to the heart [in Philo the penis and the heart are linked through reproduction] ... The fourth, and most important, that which relates to the provision thus made for prolificness.[9]
> (Philo 1993b, SL I: 4–7)

It is not that non-circumcised men do not produce sufficient seed; rather, wrote Philo, the seed gets caught in the folds of the foreskin, much as WHO doctors suggest the HIV virus does. Philo went on to write that circumcision also serves as a symbol of "the excision of the pleasures which delude the mind" and "of a man's knowing himself and discarding that terrible disease, the vain opinion of the soul" (Philo 1993c, SL II: 9). His justification for circumcision was that the rite/medical procedure corrected the body, heart and mind of the male/masculine.

For Philo, then, circumcision prevented disease, purified the body, purified the heart and ensured prolific reproduction; while penile circumcision was an outward sign that represented a likewise circumcised heart, one that was tempered, just and compassionate. Circumcision, along with tempering the heart, cooled the mind ensuring that bodily pleasures never overtook the circumcised male. As Nina Livesey has written, Philo justifies circumcision as a rite that warrants safeguarding because of its benefits for the body (I 4–7) and soul (I 9–10) (Livesey 2007, 59). Philo also contended, in his defense of circumcision, that it was a rite practiced by many peoples, including the highly respected Egyptians, along with "Arabs, and Ethiopians, and nearly all the nations who live in the southern parts of the world down to the torrid zone" (Philo 1993a, QG III: 48). Purifying as circumcision was, then, Philo took it to be a sign that spoke of the ability of the male/masculine to engage in right relations with the deity.[10]

The suggestion in the texts of Philo is that the pain of circumcision is a necessary pain to endure in order to secure the benefits that flow from it. The pain that circumcised infants/youths/adults experienced was a small price in order to secure health of the body, mind, heart, and soul, and to secure formative reproductive powers. In Judaism circumcision put the male in a right relationship with the deity and his community as it removed "the skin of the prepuce," which "is quite superfluous for generation, and is moreover especially injurious by reason of the disease of inflammation which burns with it, so also an over abundance of desire is as superfluous as it is pernicious, superfluous because it is not necessary, and pernicious because it is the cause of diseases to both body and soul" (Philo 1993a, QG: 48).

In Philo, if circumcision purifies then certainly the foreskin is impure and as such abject, a filth that incubates disease and corrupting desire: it is better to remove it for the health of the Jewish male (Boyarin 1992, 486). The pain of circumcision, although remarked upon by Philo, was nothing compared to the future pain that being uncircumcised entailed.

The writings of Josephus (37–100 CE) also discuss the issue of circumcision. In the *Life of Josephus*, the author writes that he does not feel it necessary for those who reside among the Jews to be circumcised (Josephus 1895, *Vita* 28). *Antiquities of the Jews*, however, relates the tale of Mattathias, a significant figure of the Maccabee rebellion (167–160 BCE) who:

> Overthrew their idol altars, and slew those that broke the laws, even all that he could get under his power; for many of them were dispersed among the nations round about them for fear of him. He also commanded that those boys which were not yet circumcised should be circumcised now; and he drove those away that were appointed to hinder their circumcision.
>
> (Josephus 1895, AJ 12: 268)

Circumcision was required by the law and those Jews who did not comply were made to comply by Mattathias, something the Josephus text did not directly comment on, suggesting he too considered the necessity of circumcision for Jews. Further on in *Antiquities* the author relates another story, this time concerning King Izates of Parthian who had converted to Judaism but had not been circumcised. Confronted by a wise Jew:

> "Thou dost not consider, O king! that thou unjustly breakest the principal of those laws, and art injurious to God himself, [by omitting to be circumcised]; for thou oughtest not only to read them, but chiefly to practice what they enjoin thee. How long wilt thou continue uncircumcised? But if thou hast not yet read the law about circumcision, and dost not know how great impiety thou art guilty of by neglecting it, read it now." When the king had heard what he said, he delayed the thing no longer …
>
> (Josephus 1895, AJ 20: 38)

The narrative suggests that Josephus, like Paul and Philo, took circumcision as a necessary rite to mark those who are properly Jewish. Where Philo tries to convince his reader, Josephus drew on the strong stories of the Maccabee rebellion to insist upon the rite for those who claim the identity of Jew. Equally when Josephus wrote concerning conversion to Judaism, again he insisted upon the necessity of circumcision to approach the deity of the Jews. The king was in a state of impiety and therefore an offense to the deity.

To be a Jewish man, and a good Jewish man, required the foreskin, that which offended the deity, be removed. The removal, however, registers no pain in the texts of Josephus. Infant, youth or adult, the indexical sign of pain is absent in the texts of Josephus. As in the Pauline texts, circumcision registers identity and in this register pain is a cost one must pay in order to take up the identity. Circumcision marked a relationship between deity and Jew, but also, and just as importantly, between Jew and Jew. The indexical sign of pain signifies in its absence, and in one signification as a sacrificial event, an event when the sacrifice willing gives itself over to the deity. Unregistered pain was woven into Jewish identity of the time.

In the writings attributed to these three significant Jewish figures—Paul, Philo, and Josephus—male circumcision is discussed, but the pain that accompanies it is absent or muted. Instead, circumcision serves as an identity marker of Jewishness, as a necessary physical state to approach the deity, a benefit for health and reproduction and a necessary sacrifice with a blood and flesh offering made to the deity. The indexical sign of pain, the cut, the blood, and the foreskin fall away from the concept of circumcision and are replaced with purity and deity—the gifts the writings of Philo and Josephus linked to circumcision. In Paul the ritual of circumcision falls away as a required mark to enter a relationship with the deity and baptism is proposed as a substitute rite. Both rites have their place with circumcision properly marking those who are Jews and baptism marking those who are non-Jews, even as both groups took up devotion to the deity in the Pauline texts (see also Eilberg-Schwartz 1994, 230).[11]

Text Four—Genesis, Exodus, and Joshua: The Tanakh, circumcision, and pain

The cultural Greekification of the Mediterranean, known as Hellenization, shaped the Pauline, Philoic and Josephean texts. Existential and metaphysical concerns prominent throughout the period of time (c.323 BCE–64 CE), such as the notions of salvation and a heavenly sphere, are reflected in the texts, but equally texts of the *Tanakh* are also referenced. Several texts in particular, along with their protagonists, raise the subject of circumcision locating it as a necessary rite established by the deity in the texts. Narratives found in the texts of Genesis, Exodus and Joshua locate circumcision as central to purity and related to purity, proper relationships with the deity. Proper relations with the deity secured through circumcision ensured robust reproduction (see also Eilberg-Schwartz 1994, 141) and success in warfare. The cut, the indexical sign of pain, the blood, and the foreskin were sacrificial offerings represented as desired by the deity.

Genesis 17 is typically dated to the Babylonian exile, which would be around 597–538 BCE, and is attributed to the Priestly source (Carr 2011, 292–297), although Matthew Thiessen has argued that Genesis 17 is later and should be dated to the early post-exilic period (2011, 40). As Genesis is significantly concerned with the reproductive potential secured through a contract with the deity and less concerned with identity, the latter something significant to the post-exilic period, my inclination is to take Genesis 17 to be an exilic text.

Genesis 17 provides a narrative of the protagonist Abram, who, upon having circumcised himself and all males connected to him, at the behest of the deity, was renamed Abraham. The protagonist of the text, Abram, is presented as an older male whose capacity to reproduce appears to be in question, as are the reproductive capacities of his equally aged wife Sarai. With divine intervention secured through male circumcision, however, the renamed Sarah and Abraham conceive and have a son Isaac.[12] The sealing of the contract between the deity and Abraham in the text comes in two steps: the sacrifice of the flesh of the foreskin, with more foreskins promised to the deity on a regular basis by future male descendants all on the eighth day of their lives (Gen. 17:9-16)[13] and the later preempted sacrifice of Isaac to the deity, the son of Abraham's circumcision. At the center of the contract between the deity and Abraham and his and Sarah's descendants was the sacrifice of flesh and blood, and the cut tracing the indexical sign of pain, all of which secured the reproductive potential of Sarah, Abraham, and their descendants. The indexical sign of pain, traced by the cut, is absent in the text, suggesting that the pain of the cut carried no signification. However, rather than assume no signification, its absence could be telling insofar as circumcision on the eighth day is expressed as the ideal by the deity of the text, and it may well be, then, that infant pain did not register for the author(s) of the text. This is not surprising in light of the practice of exposing infants in the marketplace in the ancient world (Boswell 1984).

The male adults and older children such as Ishmael, son of Abram by Sarai's Egyptian servant Hagar, and Abraham himself at ninety-nine years, were all circumcised upon the deity's request. The text makes no comment on the cut or the trace of pain left in the wake of circumcision, while the ritual process of the circumcision is unwritten. In the text the act is carried out expeditiously suggesting that this collective circumcision was not the proper ritual; rather Abraham and company's circumcision corrected the problematic situation of being uncircumcised in the face of the interaction between the deity and Abram. Hurriedly, then, and without comment in the text all are circumcised and, as Abraham, now a seer in close relationship with the deity, must ensure the deity's instructions are immediately acted upon. The ritual is not the one the deity in the text desires, infant circumcision, as the circumcision of youth entering manhood was practiced by other people whom the deity wanted no interaction with. Matthew Thiessen argues that the Genesis 17 requirement of eight days "moves the circumcised Ishmael to a place of liminality":

> Even more to the point, by distinguishing between Ishmael's circumcision and Isaac's, the author stresses the distance between the infant circumcision practiced by Israel and the pubescent or adult circumcision of all the other nations in the Ancient Near East that practice the rite.
> (Thiessen 2011, 41)

Howard Eilberg-Schwartz, commenting on Genesis 17, noted the shift to the practice of infant circumcision but argues it, like other pubescent circumcision, is a fertility rite (Eilberg-Schwartz 1990, 143–149) insofar as the deity's pledge to make Abraham "father of nations." Notably, however, whether infant, adolescent or adult the pain of circumcision is elided in the text.

If the text of Genesis 17 relates how the first patriarch and his kin took up the rite of infant male circumcision, the text of Exodus continues the narrative of circumcision as the rite that secures proper relations with the deity, which then ensures political, social, and economic success. The text of Exodus is layered and different sections are ascribed to different sources, but the section that interests this genealogy is Exodus 4:24-26, which is considered to be a non-priestly source, although certainly used by the priestly source to contribute to the Moses narrative (Carr 2011, 118, 289). David Carr, among others, considered the non-priestly source in question to have been contemporary with the priestly source, both of which date to the exilic and early post-exilic periods (ibid., 303).

A central protagonist of the Exodus text, Moses, is said to have been born among the oppressed Israelites of Egypt. Moses's story begins with the declaration of the Egyptian King that "every boy that is born to the Hebrews you shall throw into the Nile, but you shall let every girl live" (Ex. 1:22). In fear, the infant Moses was placed in a basket and then placed in the river by his sister and mother, whereupon the King's daughter found the infant. Wet nursed by his mother, the protagonist Moses grew to adulthood as an Egyptian, but this ended when he protected his non-Egyptian kin by killing an Egyptian. Moses fled the wrath of the pharaoh and ending up in Midian married Tsipporah (also Zipporah) and together they have two sons. While shepherding his flocks Moses was called to serve the deity. Although resisting the role the deity desired him to play, Moses finally agreed to lead the Hebrews out of Egypt. Having been called by the deity, Moses left Midian with his family and on first night of their journey they are attacked by the same deity who called him to lead the Hebrews from their slavery. Intent upon killing Moses it is only the blood and the flesh of the young son of Moses that appeases his wrath:

> On the way, at a place where they spent the night, the Lord, meet him and tried to kill him. But Zipporah took a flint and cut off her son's foreskin and touched his feet with it, and said, "Truly you are a bridegroom of blood to me." So he let him alone. It was then she said "A bridegroom of blood by circumcision."
> (Exodus 4:24-26)

Some have read this passage to mean that Moses was uncircumcised and therefore in a problematic state to interact with the deity (see Judith Sanderson, editor of Exodus in Coogan 2001, 189). Others have argued that it is unclear whose feet are meant by "his feet": the murderous deity, the protagonist Moses, or the circumcised child whose cut, blood, and foreskin warded off the rage of the deity (Talbot 2017, 206). The passage is ambivalent and polyvalent, but to simplify things only two characters act in the text: the deity and Tsipporah. It is the deity who sought to kill and Tsipporah who acted quickly and warded off the offended, and therefore, murderous deity. Warding off the deity with the sacrificial foreskin suggests that the foreskin was placed at the feet of the deity, and not Moses, as they are the actors in the section of the text.

The figure of Tsipporah in the Moses mythology is significant in this moment of the text insofar as she raises the specter of blood and flesh, and their beneficial aspects helpful to ward off a threatening deity. This notion is presented again in the text of Exodus when the blood of the sacrifice is used to mark the lintels and door posts of the Hebrews in order that the deity not visit death upon these houses (Ex. 12:23).[14] Blood is referenced twice in Tsipporah's ritualized speech and in both instances blood marked relationships: between Tsipporah and the deity; between Tsipporah and her child; and between the deity and the child. Even as the three relationships are marked, the indexical sign of pain, the cut, that joins them is absent in the text.[15] It was Tsipporah's use of a flint knife that served to reaffirm the necessity of circumcision to be in right relationship to the deity, and who emphasize the importance of the blood and foreskin of circumcision. That Tsipporah and her son entered a relationship with the deity via the cut, the blood and the foreskin is readable as a relationship of sacrifice; wherein Tsipporah offers up the pain of her child and the bloody foreskin, possibly a substitution for Moses, but certainly for the child himself, neither of whom Tsipporah was willing to deliver over to the deity.

The text of Joshua is dated to the late seventh century BCE, although sections like 5:2-12 may be indebted to earlier eighth century BCE Northern Kingdom precursors (Carr 2011, 480). The text of Joshua is a war book, and within it Joshua, not Moses, acts as military leader and warrior of the Israelites. In Joshua 5:2-12 the deity once again requests that the male Israelites be circumcised, and, as with Tsipporah, it is to be done with a flint knife: at that time the Lord said to Joshua, "take flint knives and circumcise the Israelites a second time. So Joshua made flint knives and circumcised the Israelites at Gibeath-haaraloth" (or "hill of foreskins") (Josh. 5:3). The text then explains the necessity of the commandment indicating that the second generation of those who came out of Egypt had not be circumcised and this problem needed to be rectified if the promised lands were to be acquired (Josh. 5:4-7). The mass circumcision, and the need to heal from it, was followed by the celebration of Passover. It is at this juncture the Israelites eat the produce of the land and no longer consume the "manna" that had been provided by the deity (5:10-12). The mass circumcision event of the text required that the male Israelites "remain in their places in camp until they were healed" (Josh. 5:8) registering the physical cost of circumcision and indirectly the indexical sign of pain. Genesis 34, is another narrative that proposes mass circumcision and it too registers the pain that accompanies circumcision. In Genesis 34 narrative, Dinah, the daughter of Jacob, is abducted and raped. Her brothers, seeking revenge, trick her rapist and his people into thinking they would allow the rapist to marry Dinah if he and his warriors were circumcised. Agreeing to the circumcision "on the third day, when they were still in pain, two of the sons of Jacob, Simeon, and Levi, Dinah's brothers, took their swords and came against the city unawares, and killed all the males" (Gen. 34: 25).

Both mass circumcisions registered the indexical sign of pain, pain that debilitated warriors leaving the people vulnerable. In these narratives, the cut that traces the sign of pain signified vulnerability, a problem for proper warrior masculinity. In the Joshua text, however, that vulnerability was safeguarded by the presence of the deity until the time, after Passover, the warriors were able to resume their role. In Genesis 34, however, the enfeebled warriors of Shechem are slaughtered and its inhabitants enslaved (25-29). In both narratives the cut, pain, the blood and flesh are attached to male warriors—those who are sacrificed on the field of war[16]—suggesting a sacrificial dedication, willingly given in the Joshua 5 narrative and deceitfully taken in the Genesis 34 narrative.[17] Circumcision in the text of Joshua, although weakening warriors initially, purifies and strengthens them allowing them to fight alongside the army of the deity. Allied with the deity and his army, Joshua and the Israelites take the city of Jericho (5:13-21), whereupon all the city's occupants, human and non-human animals, were sacrificed to the deity (5:21). As Thomas Römer wrote:

> The book of Joshua appropriates several concepts and ideologies of NeoAssyrian and other ancient Near Eastern warfare propaganda. Joshua's encounter with the commander of Yhwh's army can be related to Assyrian oracles in which the king receives the promise of divine assistance before the battle. In its present context, the scene follows the circumcision of the second wilderness generation and the celebration of the first Passover in the land. The divine warrior appears, therefore, after the accomplishment of rituals that highlight Israel's status as Yhwh's people.
>
> (Römer 2014, 60)

The circumcision event in Joshua 5 is linked to the success of the warfare to come. That is, to ensure their success sacrifices must be made and the foreskin of the Israelite male warrior was an ideal sacrifice to the war deity in the text of Joshua. As Römer has noted, the war angel of the deity appears to Joshua after he had circumcised his warriors having provided, then, the initial blood sacrifice that allowed the power of deity to infuse the Israelite warriors. When the circumcised warriors were victorious they then put to the sword every living being as sacrifice to the deity (Josh. 6:21).

The texts of Genesis, Exodus, and Joshua speak to the rite of male circumcision each developing and/or deploying it differently. As an indexical sign of pain, the cut signifies a relationship; that is a covenant, with the deity made on the bodies of infants (Gen. 17) and the bodies of male warriors (Josh. 5). The male infant and the male warrior are dedicated to the deity and that dedication is inscribed on their flesh. The relationship, however, is fraught since deities are dangerous and liable to turn on their adherents as much as on their enemies. It was the cut, the indexical sign of pain, blood and flesh sacrifice that protected them. The sacrifice of the foreskin and the blood of the wound also act as substitutions and provide the deity with a little of the flesh and blood of those who had been dedicated to the deity: the male infant and the warrior.

The myths of Abraham, Moses, and Joshua link each of the protagonists to the deity via the act of circumcision, while circumcision itself is represented as a means for the deity's theophany. In Genesis 17:1 the deity appears and speaks directly to Abraham, in Exodus 4:24 deity met and attacked Moses and his family, while in Joshua 5:1 the deity speaks to Joshua to request circumcision, and then again post circumcision when Joshua approached Jericho and met the warrior deity and his angelic army (Josh. 5:13). Circumcision was the rite that put the specific member of the group in relationship with the deity, but it also marked them as a sacrifice to the deity, a sacrifice that is paid in full upon the death of those who had offered their foreskins.

If the cut of circumcision acts as an indexical sign, so too does the pain of the cut. In Genesis 17:12 the direction to circumcise male infants at eight days old establishes a ritual trajectory into an unknown and distance future; Likewise, the pain that accompanies circumcision as it too will extend into eternity. The cut, the pain and the foreskin mark a relationship between the deity and the circumcised. Offering the blood, foreskin and pain to the deity secured a future for Abraham and his descendants down the long years of the deity's creation. Circumcision and the indexical sign of pain traced in the cut served to mark this eternal covenant.

Within Exodus 4 the necessity of the offering of blood and flesh, an offering wrapped in pain, is emphasized: without proper ritual, circumcision in this instance, relations between the deity and humans cannot be sustained. The deity of necessity kills the human unless the deity is properly propitiated, as the text's hero Tsipporah understood when she quickly provided the deity with the penile flesh, and blood and the pain of her male child. The deity might well have taken Moses, the child or all of them as sacrificial offerings had she not acted so quickly. Certainly Deuteronomy 12:31 and 18:10 represent the deity as rejecting child sacrifice, as that which worshipers of other deities do, but it is not necessarily the practice that is the problem; it is worshipping other deities and engaging in their ritual practices that is problematic, as Deuteronomy 13 makes clear. Equally, ritual sacrifice of human beings is certainly the outcome of the taking of Jericho wherein "they devoted to destruction by the edge of the sword all in the city; both women and men, young and old, oxen, sheep and donkeys (Josh. 7:21) suggesting then that the sacrifice of humans is not an anathema to the deity of the text. However, if not an anathema to the deity in the text it certainly may well have been problematic for humans who resist and instead substitute a small part of the ritual sacrifice, the foreskin and the blood of the cut, rather than the whole of the sacrifice, at least for the offering's lifetime. Upon death, the deity then gathers up the rest of that which was pledged: Males of Israel were the promised sacrifice, pledged in pain and fulfilled in death.

The pledging of self to the deity is a ritual act that makes sense for warriors entering the field of battle. Circumcising the flesh of the penis, as a rite of passage into warriorhood, established a link between the deity, often a warrior deity, the kind of deity represented as appearing to Joshua on the road to Jericho (5:13-15). Wielding a sword and claiming command of a divine army, the deity as warrior appears to Joshua once all the Israelite warriors have been circumcised. A blood and flesh contract, sealed with pain and blood, had been struck, the outcome of which was victory for the Israelites who survived, while those who succumbed to the sword in battle fulfilled their circumcision pledge. The pledge of the infant through the sacrifice of the foreskin and embracing pain, placed the male child under the auspices of the deity, who would collect the debt upon death.

Both kinds of male circumcision, infant and warrior, and the pain that accompanies them act as indexical signs that speak of contracts, identity, pledges, and a future down through the ages. They also internally signify shifts in the texts themselves as circumcision is made to painfully speak in numerous ways, but all the ways insist on the penis as a site of interest to the deity of the text. In Genesis male reproductive and generative potential of the penis must be attended to by the deity; in Exodus the foreskin rightly belongs to the deity as a sacrificial offering, while in Joshua warriors offered their foreskins upon which they could join the angelic army who ensured their success.

Text Five—Ancient Egypt and Circumcision as a Rite of Passage

Moses, the deliverer of the oppressed descendants of Abraham, Isaac, and Joseph from the Egyptians was questionably circumcised: that is, the myths of Moses do not speak of his circumcision either as a Hebrew or an Egyptian. The fifth-century BCE Greek historian Herodotus related in his histories: "The Egyptians and those who have learned it from them are the only people who practice circumcision" (1926, 2: 36); that "[t]hey practice circumcision for cleanliness' sake; for they would rather be clean than more becoming" (ibid., 2: 37); and that "they are the first, along with the Colchians and the Ethiopians, to practice this rite" (ibid., 2: 104). Scholars are not convinced all Egyptians practiced circumcision and some scholars suggest that only priests employed circumcision, along with the shaving off of body hair, to secure purification so as to attend the deities (Nunn 1996, 169–170; Sauneron 2000, 37–38). There does appear to be evidence, however, that circumcision was employed as a rite of passage for young men in the Old Kingdom and most likely in the pre-dynastic period. Evidence for circumcision is derived from reliefs dated to the fifth and sixth dynasties and again in the first intermediate period.

Drawing on reliefs from tombs images and texts, Ann Macy Roth has convincingly argued that the circumcision of pubescent males was a rite that allowed them to join their "phyles" (Roth 1991, 66), phyles being a social system of organization that possibly emerged in the archaic period, although there is no evidence of its existence until the first dynastic period (3000–2686 BCE). Roth speculates the phyle social systems in Egypt may well have been an aspect of social organization in general, while entrance into a phyle was secured through the rite of circumcision (ibid., 74). She conjectures that a series of ritual activities; grooming, athletics, and games related to the ridicule of deformity could well be connected to circumcision, all of which allowed the ritual participants to join their phyle (ibid., 70).

There is also significant evidence of rites of circumcision during the first intermediate period wherein a stele from Naga ed-Der has its author claiming to have been circumcised with 120 boys (Roth 1991, 71), while other monuments, all coming from Dendera, refer to people who circumcised youth and as such acted beneficently toward them (ibid., 71). Mohamed Megahed and Hana Vymazalová's study from the pyramid complex in Djedkare date it to the fifth dynasty (2494–2345 BCE). Fragments of reliefs from the tomb show two young boys who are in the process of being circumcised (Megahed and Vymazalova 2011, 156). There is also attestation of infant circumcision in the New Kingdom period (1580–1069 BCE) (ibid.).

How widespread the rite of circumcision was is unclear, but Steven Quirke argues male circumcision was widespread if not universal (2015, 49). Whether for priestly purification, for all males as a rite of passage, or for both, depending on the historical period, male circumcision is attested in ancient Egypt as early as the fifth dynasty, but the general consensus is it was practiced as early as the archaic period:

> Even though male circumcision was practised in Egypt from the predynastic times, very little direct evidence about the operation itself is available from the millennia of Egyptian history. The reliefs and statues showing both noble and lower classes of the society circumcised, and physical mummified remains from all periods of the Egyptian history indicate that circumcision was generally practiced among the Egyptian population.
> (Megahed and Vymazalová 2011, 156)

The indexical pain traced by the cut of circumcision is present in the ancient Egyptian reliefs and texts that reference the rite itself. The Old Kingdom examples from fifth- and sixth-dynasty tomb reliefs depict the act of cutting the head of the penis with those receiving the cut requiring calming or assistance during the rite. In the fifth dynasty relief of the Djedkare tomb complex two young boys are being circumcised and behind them is a woman with spread arms encircling the boys in a gesture of reassurance. In the sixth-dynasty tomb relief of ʿnh-m-ʿHr the circumcisee is held from behind by another man, while the circumciser holds the penis in one hand and in his other hand is the instrument that is posed to cut the penis (Roth 1991, 67). The caption above the image reads "Hold him fast; do not let him fall!" (Nunn 1996, 169). On the stele from Naga ed-Der dated to the first intermediate period, the circumcised youth indicated that he nor any of his group of 120 ritual participants scratched or hit anyone while being cut. All three of the references to circumcision register the pain that comes with the cut, and indeed represent the circumcised engaging the indexical sign traced by the cut.

In the Old Kingdom reliefs there is no sense of the circumcised needing to endure the pain stoically and instead there is an expectation that the circumcisee may well succumb to the pain. If, as Roth and others have argued, the relief depicts the circumcision of sons of a priest, the young men who ritually prepared to take up the role of a ka-priest in order to attend their father's tomb upon his death (Roth 1991, 66), then ritual purity is more than likely the effort and result of the cut. The indexical sign of pain is an inescapable aspect of the purification rite. Pain comes with the circumcision and is a necessary part of the rite be it absent or present. The circumcision of the 120 male youths, with its reference to the capacity of author of the Naga ed-Der stele to endure pain, marks its presence. Circumcision of the penis appears to have included a test of bravery, at least in the mind of Wḥ3 the author of the stele. He, like his compatriots, showed themselves to be no longer male children but adults in their capacity to endure the cut.

In the Egyptian reliefs, eight-day-old male infants are not represented as those circumcised, although certainly infant circumcision was practiced in the New Kingdom. Rather, male youths are represented as those circumcised, and furthermore, these youth are represented as encountering pain when circumcised. The pain of circumcision is not absent and indeed is present as the text signifies its unavoidability, in the case of the ka-priest purification rite ("hold him fast lest he fall") and its necessity to be overcome in the rite of passage into a phyle and adulthood. The indexical sign of pain traced by the cut signifies strongly in the texts remarking on its relationship to the bodies of Egyptian male children and youth.

Observations and Insights

Tracking circumcision back through to the Old Kingdom of ancient Egypt one can see how it has been, as an indexical sign, made to carry multiple significations some of which appear to have been associated with the rite from its earliest known practice and have been carried up through the ages. This carry forward is not a situation of an unbroken line; rather, meanings surface, disappear and resurface. Purity, for example, is one such signification appearing as it does in all of the texts of this genealogical endeavor, albeit how purity means shifts depending on the text. In ancient Egypt purity is a physical state one needed to be in to approach deities. In Joshua and Exodus, a state of purity is also suggested and equally suggested is the necessity to be in this state to approach the deity. Circumcising as a means to achieve a state purity appears as well in the Philoic text but does not appear in the Josephean or the Pauline texts. Once we enter the modern period we see that purity again surfaces as a significant meaning of circumcision in the nineteenth, twentieth, and twenty-first centuries. In these texts, however, purity does not signify a state of being required to approach the deity; rather circumcision moved the male youth into a proper moral state, one that was acceptable to the social body and would ensure his well-being. Scroll forward to the twenty-first century and the HIV/AIDS global epidemic, once again purity is signified; the purity of the social body and the human body. Circumcising and purifying black African penises is meant to purify the larger social body from HIV/AIDS.

Infant, youth and adult male circumcision, the indexical sign of pain, appear in many social and historical locations signifying in a multitude of ways, but all of which seek to reshape masculinity just as the flint, knife, razor, or scalpel reshaped the penis. The cut, an indexical sign that signifies the passage of pain, brings echoes of the Belgian Congo where so many Congolese lost their lives. Reshaping the penis of the black African male under the auspices of the WHO brings echoes of Rudyard Kipling's "White Man's Burden." In countries throughout sub-Saharan and Eastern Africa millions of boys, youth, and men are being circumcised in order to stay the spread of HIV/AIDS. Removing that which is envisioned as collecting disease, the foreskin signifies as abject and must be removed before it contaminates the rest of the body, while the body when contaminated threatens to contaminate the entirety of the specific social body and the contamination of the specific social body the contamination of the global body.

The foreskin as a thing of abjection is also an aspect of the necessity to circumcise in general throughout the late nineteenth century and early twentieth century in the US and Canada. Circumcision to correct diseases of the body, mind and spirit was wholeheartedly embraced by social engineers, doctors of the body and mind, and the Christian religious. The excess flesh on the head of the penis threatened not only the body of the male, but his mind and soul as well. Staring down the barrel of masturbatory madness, the young male must be curbed and shaped appropriately in-line with the operative masculinity. The foreskin was thought to increase sexual pleasure leaving the male open to a wanton desire that produced lascivious behavior. The foreskin's removal and the indexical sign of pain, the cut, act to squelch any excessive sexual desire: indeed, the passage of pain was the whip seen to curb sexual desire. The foreskin is once again the abject that must be cast aside. It is tainted by its own excess and that excess is sexual desire. If the male is not circumcised he is or will be improperly masculine and therefore subject to excessive desire. Subject to his excessive desire he cannot dominate and instead will be dominated. The foreskin, left attached to the penis, disempowered the male leaving him open to disease, the morally suspect, and ultimately meant a return to an earlier state in evolution, when the human was more an animal. The cut propelled the male from a state of nature to a civilized state, while the pain marked the passage from one way of being to the next. Properly civilized, the circumcised male is properly masculine allowing him to take up his proper place in the world.

Moving on to the Greco-Roman texts reflecting Hellenistic systems of belief and practice, identity is emphasized in the Pauline and Josephean texts which represent circumcision as a necessary rite for those who live within the covenant of Abraham and the law of Moses. In the Pauline texts, the rite is unnecessary for those who access the spirit of Jesus Christ through baptism. The Pauline texts propose that the rite of circumcision replaces the rite of baptism for non-Jews who wish to share in the blessings of Abraham (Gal. 3:14). The rite of circumcision acted as a blood and flesh offering that indexically marked the infant as belonging to the deity and the deity's people. The flow of blood, the sacrifice of the foreskin and the pain signified the beginning of a relationship between the infant, the community and the deity in Judaism. The rite of baptism and possession by the spirit—"Now we have received not the spirit, but the spirit that is from God, so that we may understand the gifts bestowed on us by God. And we speak of these things in words not taught by human wisdom but taught by the Spirit interpreting spiritual things to those who are spiritual" (1 Cor. 2:12-13)—redefined the ritual means by which to enter into a contract with the deity.

The texts of Philo, like those of Josephus and Paul, take circumcision to mark those operating within the covenant of Abraham and the laws of Moses, but Philo, in defense of the rite, provided a number of aspects that further flesh out the indexical sign. The Philoic texts did not see the rite as painless, however the pain and blood where necessary in order to achieve the proper state of purity wherein the foreskin was removed. The circumcised penis, wrote Philo, ensured the health of the body, and opened the way to achieve a properly circumcised heart, mind, and soul as prescribed by the laws of Moses.

The texts of Genesis 17, Exodus 4, and Joshua 5 engage the rite of circumcision. Genesis 17 provides the origin myth for the rite, although the pain is made absent at this moment of origin. The rite is a covenant of flesh and blood the outcome of which is the offering of the foreskin, a pledge that speaks to a later offering of the whole self. In the text, the protagonist Abraham presumably circumcised himself, and, like the Egyptian deity Re in the Book of the Dead,[18] he does not succumb to the pain. The absence of a register of pain signals both a disregard for pain even as it signals a capacity to endure pain; in Genesis 17 a pain necessary to achieve reproductive potential. The indexical sign of reproductive prowess, circumcision, signifies a reproductive covenant between the deity, Abraham, and Sarah wherein their line will multiple and live forward in an eternal future.

Circumcision as the sign of a reproductive covenant fades into the background when the protagonist of Exodus, Moses, enters a relationship with the deity on behalf of Abraham's descendants. The sign's meaning has shifted to emphasize covenant, agreement, and loyalty to the deity, a signification that is emphasized in the story of the attack by the deity upon the company of Moses. The blood and flesh secured by Tsipporah's deft cut of her son acted to ward off the deity's intent to kill. Receiving or perceiving the bloody foreskin, the deity departs assuaged by the blood and flesh offering. The blood of circumcision foreshadows the lamb's blood on the lintel and doorposts of the Hebrews when the deity strikes the first-born males of Egypt, while both rites, now connected in the narrative of Exodus, are to be practiced in perpetuity (Ex. 12:23-24). The deity's murderous attack on Moses's company and deity's murderous attack on first born males are deflected by circumcision, a necessary rite for males to participate in the Passover (Ex. 12:48). In the text, the cut, the flesh, and the blood are a promissory offering of the whole to come later upon the death of the circumcised. Through circumcision every male is redeemed, while upon their deaths each pays their debt to the deity.

The text of Joshua replaces Moses with Joshua, who is depicted as leading the Israelites into war. The deity of the text of Joshua requires that all the males be circumcised—with no age directive provided. The eight day circumcision requirement imposed on Abraham is absent and instead all the males are mass circumcised and given three days to heal, whereupon they celebrate Passover, once more linking blood and flesh of the circumcision with the blood of the sacrifice that marked the lintel and door posts. The pain of circumcision is acknowledged in the texts, but the pain of the warriors is assuaged by the Passover. They recover their strength and now purified march with the deity's angelic army. In Joshua, circumcision purifies allowing the Israelite warriors to march with the deity; but equally marked each as a sacrificial offering. Two significations of the indexical sign of pain, the cut, are purification and a promissory offering of a bit of abject flesh.

Circumcision as a mark of purification plays out in ancient Egypt, the site of the earliest evidence for the rite. The rite of circumcision, along with shaving the body, was a necessity in order that priests approach their deities (Megahed and Vymazalova 2011, 158-159). Purity was a state achieved by the removal of all potential sites of the accumulation of dirt and vermin that would pollute the temples of the deities. But others beside priests practiced the rite of passage traced by the cut seen on tomb walls from the Old Kingdom and the intermediate period. In these cases, scholars have argued that circumcision was necessary to take up adult status, most likely in a phyle. In these texts the indexical sign of pain traced by the cut is given presence as something that must be endured and overcome in order to achieve the state needed; purity or adulthood both achieved by the shedding of the blood of the penis.

The indexical sign of pain registered by the cut, has multiple significations with some of the more persistent being purity and identity, while cleanliness is often linked with purity and turns up almost as frequently. The WHO's efforts to halt the spread of HIV/AIDS locates the foreskin and circumcision in a discourse of medical purity, one that includes circumcision as cleansing, that disregards any reference to pain, but pain is present and its erased passage signifies a colonial relationship of oppression wherein the uncircumcised black penis threatens global health and so must be attended to. As black male hypersexuality is curbed by the indexical sign of pain, the cut, so too the threat of pubescent male masturbation and their potential hypersexuality. The cut, again deployed in medical discourse, prevented such possibilities and served to purify the body and mind of the male child, who might like those others, including the female feminine, succumb to their desires. In the twentieth century the narrative was stepped up with moral purity replaced by physical purity, which then was linked to overall well-being. The male infant is cut, while his cries of pain are denied much like the pain of non-human animals is denied. The blood and flesh of the infant is wiped away and discarded, while the indexical sign, the cut and the pain that attends the cut, signify of the child's entrance into human relations—an entrance marked by their denied pain. The cut in the texts of Philo, Exodus and Joshua signifies purity, the purity necessary to approach the deity and to carry out the deity's demands, a signification found in the Egyptian texts as well. Found in the ancient Egyptian texts was an extension of purity to include cleanliness, something Philo took to be a benefit of the cut as well. The circumcised penis signified the state of purity of those who bore the mark.

The cut as a mark of identity appears in the ancient texts examined with significant regularly. The majority of texts took circumcision to be the mark that identified those who traced their genealogy back to Abraham and who obey the laws of Moses. Paul, Philo, and Josephus took the cut to be a necessary rite in order to adhere to the laws of Moses. For Philo the indexical sign opened the path to proper relations with the deity wherein one's heart, mind, and soul were also properly circumcised. Equally so with Genesis 17, Exodus 4 and Joshua 5-6, those who are the people of the deity are those who bear the indexical sign of circumcision. Tsipporah recognized this when she circumcised her son and offered the flesh to the deity, just as Abram/Abraham and Joshua's warriors did when they offered their foreskins and blood to their deity. Finally, as a rite of passage in ancient Egypt and as the indexical sign that marks Egyptian priests, the cut marked the movement from one way of being to another: from child to adult and lay to religious. The indexical sign of pain traced in the cut carries multiple meanings, but all of these meanings are essential to the construction of maleness, adulthood, masculinity and warriors in the textual context from which they are derived. Purity, cleanliness, identity, piety, offering and sacrifice are declined in the male/masculine referencing as they do the penis/phallus. For the warriors of the deity the penis and sword were unsheathed and ready to do battle, while for the eight-day-old infant the cut and pain are but an offering he provides that later will be redeemed. In these texts, the blood, the flesh, and the cut tracing the indexical sign of pain must be borne by the male/masculine in order that he might achieve his potential and a future.

Afterword

Joan Scott's pivotal text on experience argues that experience too is a social construction shaped within and by our linguistic systems:

> When experience is taken as the origin of knowledge, the vision of the individual subject (the person who had the experience or the historian who recounts it) becomes the bedrock of evidence on which explanation is built. Questions about the constructed nature of experience, about how subjects are constituted ... in the first place, about how one's vision is structured—about language (or discourse) and history—are left aside.
>
> (Scott 1991, 777)

As with experience, so too with pain. The indexical sign of pain is part of a linguistic system that serves, like sexuality, as a dense transfer point of power. At the dark site of Abu Ghraib and in the soldiers' messes of Sparta, rites wherein the flesh was scored marking the passage of the indexical sign of pain, masculinities were constructed and those who fell outside, the "Islamic terrorist" or the "trembler", lacked proper masculinity being, as it was performed, being inherently "feminine." So too in ancient biblical texts where the signification of proper warrior masculinity was defined in and through the indexical sign of pain: Those who succumbed die, while those who do not live, even if that living is only until the next battle wherein deity may well collect the promised male warrior. Like the male infant whose cut, blood and foreskin serve as a promissory note, explicitly registered in the sacrifice of Isaac or Saul's bride price of one hundred Philistine foreskins that David might marry his daughter Michal (1 Sam. 18:25), the warrior's life belongs to deity: he is a sacrifice.

The indexical sign of pain acts as an ontological truth, a truth that divides those who occupy the space of the same and those who occupy the space of the other; the infant male body, the racialized male body, the feminized male body, the sacrificial male body and the non-human animal body. Those who occupy the space of the other, unsurprisingly, are subject to censure and physical adjustment as they have been found wanting as properly masculine, adult, human or even existent. Spartan male citizens and Israelite warriors, Egyptian youths, Islamic terrorists and non-human animals find their way to definition via the indexical sign of pain. The cut of circumcision, the welt of the lash, the shock of the electrode and the gash of the knife are indexical signs of pain that have been traced upon the bodies of those who are other and/or those transiting out of the space of the other. Subject to pain, they are subject to their bodies; however, if they do not succumb to pain, then they are no longer subject to their bodies. Jeremy Wisnewski (2010, 40) wrote that "Elaine Scarry's point that torture attempts to reduce a person to his body—to the singularity of pain experienced as one's body—is correct …" What both Wisnewski and Scarry miss, however, is that we are completely and always bodies and there is no other possible ontology. Both Wisnewski and Scarry operate inside the logic of modernity wherein the prevalent ontology is a body and mind separation, one that mirrors the body and soul separation of Christianity. Christianities propose a soul that survives the death of the physical body and another space called heaven wherein existence of humans, and sometimes dogs, continues. The view assumes that humans are more than their bodies, and although I would agree humans, and all life, are more than the sum of their parts, these parts are all bodily parts, even cognition, too often touted as "mind," is utterly flesh and blood: there is no metaphysical mind.

In this work, engaging the indexical sign of pain has not only allowed me to challenge Scarry's argument that pain is "anterior" to language, but it also allows me to locate the corporal in language and language in the corporal and this then is a step in a direction away from the body and mind binary that haunts and shapes our knowledge of being in the world, of bodies, of flesh—our ontologies. The body and mind binary, along with the human animal and non-human animal binary, the feminine and masculine binary, the child and adult binary, and the same other binary, serve to continue and further oppressive systems. Following pain we see how being subject to the body signifies as problematic and marks those who succumb as lacking; lacking proper masculinity, proper humanity, and proper being. The indexical sign of pain identifies those who are not human, those who are warriors, those who are terrorists, those who are black male Africans, those who are pure, those who are Jews, those who are ka priests and the newly made men of the Egyptian phyles. Embedded in ritual or ritualized, the indexical sign of pain signifies in a multitude of ways.

Notes

Introduction

1. If one follows Jacques Lacan the preverbal stage precedes the mirror stage, which is set at about six months (Lacan 2007).

Chapter 1

1. Certainly there have been numerous articles as well, while recent studies in religion and animals have also brought the body back into the analysis (see, for example, Waldau and Patton 2006; Wolfe 2003a, 2003b; Baker 1993).
2. Binaries are also not stable and value along with meaning can shift depending on the context. For example, when nature signifies as unspoiled and devoid of cynicism and deception, the body can function as a place of truth, a premise that undergirds the logic of torture, and therefore functions as positive in binary relationship with the mind figured as deceiving and self-deceiving. For a discussion of the body as a reservoir of truth see DuBois 1991; Silverman 2001.
3. My reading of Lacan is shaped by a number of theorists, Louis Althusser (1971), Elizabeth Grosz (1990), Kaja Silverman (1983), and Chris Weedon (2001).
4. It goes without saying that often included in the object/subject binary set are nature/culture, animal/human, female/male, and savage/civilized, see Sherry Ortner (1974) or Michel de Certeau (1988, 1993). Certainly, binaries, like metaphors, metonymies, and synecdoches, are not fixed and always in flux with meaning and power shifting depending on circumstance, time and place.
5. Unlike Freud, I reject the concept of "the mind" finding it to be a construct used to privilege a few over the many based on gender, race, geopolitical location and ablebodiedness.
6. For an example of this see Freud's view of the source of the drives in a physical process ("in an organ or part of the body, whose stimulus is represented in the psyche by the drive") in "the Unconscious" (Freud 2005, §§655–660).
7. She comments that "In such a view [wherein structures or impersonal forces, such as power, construct the subject] the grammatical and metaphysical place of the subject is retained even as the candidate that occupies that place appears to rotate [e.g., "discourse constructs the subject"]. As a result, construction is still understood as a unilateral process initiated by a prior subject, fortifying that presumption of the metaphysics of the subject that where there is activity, there lurks behind it an initiating and willful subject" (Butler 1993, 9).

8. As I read Michel Foucault, neither bodies nor societies are closed systems; rather as power moves via networks, bodies, and societies themselves must be conceptually thought of as porous, shifting, and unstable with no clear boundaries.
9. Eco writes in his *A Theory of Semiotics*, "[p]roperly speaking there are not signs, but only *sign-functions* ... Therefore the classical notion of 'sign' dissolves itself into a highly complex network of changing relationships" (Eco 1979, 49, emphasis original).
10. In this quote Butler is referring to the sign of "women," but what she writes is equally applicable to the body and pain.
11. John Locke's position, however, that non-human animals did have sensory apparatus and therefore felt pain on a deep level (Locke 1975), thankfully won the day.
12. According to the *Oxford English Dictionary*, the word as applied to animals' lack of reason is used in the late fifteenth century, for example, brute beast, and as an adjective describing humans demonstrating a similar orientation in the sixteenth century and more popularly in the seventeenth century.
13. Mythemes, as I use the term, deviating somewhat from Claude Lévi-Strauss (1963, 210–211) are elemental themes or singular strands that act as aphoristic presentments that relate cultural truths. In my usage I have generalized Lévi-Strauss's definition of mythemes and although I also understand mythemes to be gross constituent units, they are units that interweave with the socio-cultural body of knowledge rather than just myths as Lévi-Strauss understood them to function. These constituent units or mythemes are often considered to be profound and/or relevant truths that are accepted, rejected, or contested within social bodies.
14. We read that although the process of scarification is not understood as a rite of passage by the community at large, Lincoln notes that young women who began and complete the process often behave as if a threshold had been crossed exhibiting pride concerning their marks particularly to those young women who lacked them. He also notes that a young man of good family is asked to cleanse the scars once they are healed, and that the scars themselves, although variable, all had a basic schemata: a line from the throat to the navel and the navel with concentric circles around it. All of this suggests, states Lincoln, that one is encountering a rite of passage, even if it has not been formalized (Lincoln 1981, 34–49).

Chapter 2

1. Neo-Darwinists such as Richard Dawkins and his text *The Ancestor's Tale* (2004) make this point even more forcefully.
2. Binary categories are not fixed with regard to value. For example, the female/male binary can change value, that is from female (–) and male (+) to the reverse, depending on the discursive context. With regard to a natural and normative

state of nurturing the young, for example, the female tends to signify positively while the male negatively as he is absent. See, for example, Chodorow (1978).
3. Binaries, as has been well demonstrated, are not universal and indeed are contextually bound and operative in a social body; see in particular Marilyn Strathern (1980) against the redevelopment by binarism of Sherry Ortner (1996).
4. In this set I used the animal/human binary as the root binary largely because many foundational myths I am aware of develop discourses to distinguish between the two. Another frequent distinction is that between female and male, which I have also treated as a root binary (see Juschka 2009).
5. The great chain of being, of course, has a history of its own and certainly understanding of the notion changes under the influence of the then current historical and social exigencies (see Lovejoy 1960, ch. 6 ff. for his historical examination of the idea).
6. There are a number of English translations of the *Popol Vuh*, but I find Dennis Tedlock's (1996) most compelling. See Denise Low (1992) for a discussion of the English translations of the *Popol Vuh* and her preference for Tedlock's translation, although not without some criticisms such as Tedlock's choice of largely prose over poetic text. I also drawn on Allen Christenson's poetic version (2004, 2007).
7. I am using episteme in the sense that Michel Foucault developed it: "I would define the episteme retrospectively as the strategic apparatus which permits of separating out from among all the statements which are possible those that will be acceptable within, I won't say a scientific theory, but a field of scientificity, and which it is possible to say are true or false. The episteme is the 'apparatus' which makes possible the separation, not of the true from the false, but of what may from what may not be characterised as scientific" (Foucault 1980b, 197).
8. This aspect can also be found in demogonic myths, but what one often finds in the demogonic myth is the employment of the anthropogonic myth that separates human and non-human animals to mark divisions within and without the group or *demos* (politico-social group).
9. A fixed version of the epics of Homer emerged after the third century BCE from the work of the Alexandrian scholars (Rutherford 1996, 19).
10. Non-human and human animal overlapping is currently how science understands non-human and human animals. See Midgley (1995) for an historical analysis of scientific and philosophical conceptualization of the boundary.
11. There are few tales of the inverse wherein animals are changed into humans and behave as humans. One that Sir J. G. Frazer refers to is attributed by the scholiast to Hesiod in his commentary on Pindar (N. 3.13(21)) wherein the Myrmidons (warriors of Achilles in the *Iliad*) are said to have been ants that Zeus changed into men to populate the empty island Aegina whose occupants had been killed by Hera who had been enraged by Zeus's infidelity with Aegina (Hyginus, Fab. 52). See also Strab. 8.6.16; and Ov. Met. 7.614 ff. for reference to this myth (Apollodorus 1961–63, 63, 3.12.6 n. 8). The *Iliad*, however, does not reference this story, although in the text the Myrmidon tend to be represented collectively. In one instance

Hermes, sent by Zeus, takes the form of a Myrmidon in order to assist Priam and guide him among the Achaeans in his effort to claim the body of his son Hector (24. 395–404).

12. Hybrid figures such as centaurs or satyrs abound in Greek myth, and certainly are referred to in the Homeric texts. These beings, however, are not a mix of the human and animal; rather, they are altogether different as they are otherworldly beings who occupy the wild space surrounding human habitations. Their otherness is signified by their tail, horn, hoof, or fur, the latter of which marks their location of place/space as wild. In other instances of hybridization where there is a mix of non-human and human animals, these figures are represented as monstrous, such as the Minotaur son of Pasiphae and Poseidon's bull. The Minotaur, housed in a labyrinth, had the head of a bull and the body of a human, ate human flesh and never spoke. In still other instances hybrids represent not a mixing of human and non-human animals, but are rather the children of deities, for example, Erichthonius, who was part snake and deity and a mythical king of Athens. Even semi-divine beings who appear to be linked to non-human animals, such as Heracles and his wardrobe of animal skins and bestial madness, are not. Heracles's non-human animal attributes signify his semi-divine status, and the risks therein, as a son of Zeus and not his kinship with the non-human animal. When it comes to non-human and human animals in the texts, bonds of kinship are not imagined and indeed what is imagined is their difference signified by lack (–).
13. I am indebted to John Heath (2005) for my discussion on animals and speech in the Homeric epics.
14. See *The Golden Ass* by Apuleius (2011) for the continuance of this idea.
15. The intent here, I think, is to mark the dead as non-human and this is rhetorically achieved by drawing upon the category of the non-human animal and their non-human speech, to mark the difference.
16. Heath writes: "The lack of language, the defining characteristic of animals in the Homeric epics, is thus redefined as an absence of authoritative speech in those who lack power. Women are born with this cultural deficiency, although some manage to work around it slightly. Men too are born deficient, but they have the chance to outgrow their weakness. In some ways, this acquisition of *muthoi* is the definition of manhood, and thus of the heroic life in general. If to die is to lose the power of speech, then the corollaries might be that to grow up is to gain it, and to live fully is to exercise it. Nowhere are these associations more clear than in the heroic ethos, where to be successful is to be a doer of deeds and speaker of words" (Heath 2005, 77).
17. In an earlier passage (2.459–464) Greeks are likened to tribes of winged birds "wild geese or cranes or long-necked swans," but in this instance cranes signify positively and represent the Greeks' strength and vast numbers, "glorying in their strength of wing, and with loud cries settle ever onwards, and the meadow resounds …"

18. John Heath (2005) has argued that it is human speech that acts as a primary criterion to mark the boundary between human and non-human animals in ancient Greece, but I would further argue that the concept of kinship—the notion of tribe—is another important criterion toward establishing this boundary as is pain, which I discuss in the next section.
19. For example, see *Iliad* 1.225, 11.317, 18.433 and *Odyssey* 1.287, 2.82, 3.209 for endure; and *Il.* 4.94, 5.21, 22.236 or *Od.* 1.257, 2.82, 2.219, 4.242, 4.445 for daring to or not. Endure is the most common meaning in the *Odyssey*, but also, on occasion to mean "suffer to" e.g., swear an oath 10.343 and "dare to" e.g., come down to Hades 11.475.
20. See also Nemesis, the abstract personification of divine justice and retribution.
21. The term turns up fourteen times in the *Iliad*, but in four instances the term refers to sorrow or pain of the heart, and six times in the *Odyssey* with four usages referring to anguish and emotional pain.
22. *Stenakhô* is also used in the *Iliad* twice to refer to a roar (16.391, 16.393) and four times in the *Odyssey* to refer to being overwhelmed by the sea (4.516, 5.420, 7.274, 23.317), while *stonoeis* is used six times to speak of arrows or missiles loaded with pain; three in each of the *Iliad* (8.159, 15.590, 17.374) and *Odyssey* (21.12, 21.60, 24.180).
23. The impact of deity on environment is dependent on the power of the deity under consideration. For example, Demeter's wrath over the abduction of her daughter was universally applied and hurt humans and non-human animals and deities, while Apollo's wrath tends to be local and hurts/helps a person or group.
24. As Petropoulos comments, the wounding above the knee refers to the "notional seat of manhood" and therefore is comparable to male circumcision (2011, 119).
25. The pattern of the textual rite follows closely Arnold van Gennep's (1960) structural model (separation, transition or liminality, and incorporation) whereby the initiate is marked and then separated from the community, seen in the naming and then journey away from Ithaka to his maternal grandfather in Parnassas. In the sea journey he is represented as occupying a transitional state, visit and hunt with maternal male/masculine relatives, that is, his grandfather and uncles. And finally, incorporation can be seen in Odysseus's successful return home whereupon, as Petropoulos notes (2011, 120), "the young man gives an eloquent account of the exploits to his rejoicing parent," marking the first of many narratives that are attached to his name over time.
26. However, even properly masculine warriors can be overcome by pain (and therefore fail in the heroic effort), but when this occurs, as in the case of the death of Sarpedon (16.486), he roars or bellows (*bebruxos*), in response to the pain and in doing so gives his death cry (s.v. Liddell and Scott 1968). Book 13. 393 of the *Iliad* uses *bebrukhe* in a similar if less dramatic fashion.
27. Also suggested in this idea of an inner self is the notion of the human "mind" that is "inside the body" seen in René Descartes, among many others, in the early modern period (Foucault 1980a; Winquist 1998).

28. The Greek term 'ιερεύω (*iereus*) is used to mean both sacrifice and slaughter in the Homeric texts (s.v. Liddell and Scott 1968).
29. For further examples see, *Il.* 6.174, 6.309, 7.314, and esp. 21.103–133; and *Od.* 11.32–33, 13.24–25, 13.181–182, 19.198.
30. A good modern example of films that make the horse central in masculine warfare is the 2011 film *War Horse* directed by Steven Spielberg.
31. The war horse is typically depicted as both male and masculine, and masculine insofar as "he" too must be willing to risk pain and death in battle. The war horse shares in the masculine heroic narrative.
32. See also *Il.* 17.475–478 when the personal identity narrative of Patroclus recites his ability to master Achilles horses in order to signify his heroic nature and therefore proper warrior masculinity (albeit briefly lived).
33. Telemachus, gifted with a chariot and three horses, turns back the gift and requests instead some other treasure. His remark is that horses are not that useful on the rocky terrain of Ithaka (*Od.* 4.600–608).
34. According to Liddell and Scott (1968), μακών occurring in the phrase κὰδ δ' ἔπεσ' ἐν κονίῃσι μακών expresses the wounding and collapsing of an animal such as a stag, horse, or boar. Note that the horse is classified with wild non-human animals in terms of the groups of non-human animals represented as dying in this fashion.
35. The name Irus is a play on the deity Iris since Irus was wont to run errands for anyone who asked (l. 5–7).
36. The traditional time-line of the Maya civilization is: Archaic 9000–2300 BCE; Early Formative 2300–900 BCE; Middle Formative 900–400 BCE; Late Formative 400 BCE–250 CE; Early Classic 250–400 CE; Middle Classic 400–550 CE; Late Classic 550–850 CE; Terminal Classic 850–1000 CE; Early Post-Classic 1000–1200 CE; and Late Post-Classic 1200–1521 CE (Joyce 2000, 3; Coe 1999).
37. See for example, part 3 of the *Popol Vuh* wherein the hero twins, Huanhpu and Xbalanque, are assisted by non-human animals allowing them to overcome the Xibablans.
38. Other K'iche' words that refer to pain found in Christenson's (2004) translation are the verb *jilowik* meaning to groan with pain; to moan; or to complain about pain on page 250, *k'aqaxuwik* referring to tooth pain found on page 40, and the noun *q'oxom* meaning pain used on page 39. *K'ax* is the word most frequently used in text to refer to pain and is found on pages 26, 28, 29, 41, 154.
39. All of them,   Ronojel,
    Were crushed their faces,   Xq'utu ki wach.
    These the stones,   Are' ri ab'aj,
    They their hearthstones,   Ri ki xk'ub',
    Would flatten them,   Chitaninik,
    Would come from fire,   Chipe pa q'aq',

Landed on their heads,	Taqal chi ki jolom,
Pain was done to them.	K'ax xb'an chike
	(Christenson 2004, 28–29)

40. Their birth narrative does not appear until part 3 of the *Popol Vuh*.

Chapter 3

1. *Homoioi* is a Spartan concept that refers to those who are peers or equals and who share the same status.
2. Gorgo is a Greek name for Gorgon (Γοργώ), particularly Medusa, whose head adorned Zeus's aegis; a protective garment or shield that was also worn by Athena his daughter. In Hesiod the famous snake-headed Medusa is the daughter of Phorkys and Keto, sister and brother, and offspring of Gaia, the earth and Pontos, the sea. One of three gorgons, her sisters are Sthenno and Euryale, it was Medusa's gaze that turned those who met it into stone. In material representation, the Gorgons were popular subjects and often appears with grotesque faces, tongues dangling out of their mouths, and bulging eyes. These representations are suggestive of the Gorgon as apotropaic—-that is driving evil away—but equally appears also to have represented the warrior's battle fury and was used to intimidate enemies. Jean-Pierre Vernant wrote, referencing Homer, that "[i]n this context of merciless confrontation, Gorgo is a Power of Terror, associated with Fear and Rout and Pursuit which chills the heart" (Vernant 1991, 117). As an adjective *gorgos* refers to "grim, fierce, terrible of look or gaze" but also appears to be linked in another form to "spirited as related to horses" (Beekes 2009, 283); an apt connection in light of Medusa's rape by Poseidon (associated with horses) and the birth of Pegasus (and the giant with the golden sword Chrysaor) from her neck when Perseus slew her.
3. Jane Carter argues for the Phoenician origin of the rites that took place at the altar of Ortheia, as well as arguing that the rites involved the *hieros gamos* within which the masks were used (Carter 1986, 1987).
4. Rosenberg's argument locates the shift from ritual drama to theatrical drama at Ortheia's altar and the rites that took place there (Rosenberg 2015, 259).
5. The *diaulos* was also played at athletic and poetic competitions as well as being played during the funeral procession to the graveside.
6. Liminality is the state of betwixt and between, the threshold concept that speaks to transition. See van Gennep (1960).
7. Ducat (2006a, 273), however, argued that all the performers in the Gymnopaidiai were naked which precludes this as evidence for the initiation of boys. I would disagree, however, arguing that rites of passage can be contained within and/or linked to other significant ritual practices. The festival of the Gymnopaidiai was clearly agonistic, as most agree, and therefore the agon would not only be for the children, but for all age classes.

8. Iphigenia was sacrificed to Artemis in order to appease her wrath allowing Agamemnon to leave for war in Troy. During the sacrificial process, however, Artemis whisked Iphigenia off to the barbaric Tauris where she served Artemis helping to sacrifice humans to her. Orestes was able to rescue Iphigenia and the two return to Sparta. Orestes was a favored of Apollo, Artemis's brother and it was Apollo who counselled Orestes to murder his mother and her lover and Apollo who assisted in clearing him of the blood guilt of these murders.

Chapter 4

1. I use the term "third world" as a means to keep in historical consciousness how colonized locations around the globe were ideological battlegrounds between the "first world" or the Eurowest and the "second world" or the Soviet Union. As I use the term, no intention of hierarchy is implied; rather the tension between dominant global powers during this period.
2. For example, in early modern France, the viability of torture as a means to secure the truth was vociferously challenged by numerous writers. Augustin Nicolas, *président* of the *parlement* of Dijon, wrote that torture produced false confessions or Sonnenfels who wrote "[i]n the critical instance in which sensibility is pushed to the extreme, pain triumphs over the accused: but what is the cry that it tears from him? That of truth? What error! ... It is really that of weakness, that speaks in a man tortured in this way" (in Silverman 2001, 161, 173). Equally, the FBI responding to the use of torture to gain information at Guantánamo wrote in a memo that such techniques "were not effective or producing [i]ntel that was reliable" (quoted in Jaffer and Singh 2007, 10). Darius Rejali (2007, 478) has written that: "In short, organized torture yields poor information, sweeps up many innocents, degrades organizational capabilities, and destroys interrogators. Limited time during battle or emergency intensifies all these problems. These results do not prove that torture never works to produce accurate information. That would misread the scientific and social scientific evidence, and, at any rate, impossibility arguments are hard to prove."
3. According to Jaffer and Singh (2007, 29) "a report issued February 2006 by Human Rights First found that nearly one hundred prisoners had died in US custody since August 2002 and of these deaths thirty-four had been classified by military investigators as suspected or confirmed homicides."
4. There has been some good subsequent analysis, some of which I am indebted to in this chapter (see for example Greenberg and Dratel 2005; Jaffer and Singh 2007; Morris 2008).
5. Included among the recommendations of the Working Group Report on Detainee Interrogations in the Global War on Terrorism: Assessment of Legal, Historical, Policy, and Operational Considerations, dated April 4, 2003, was that "techniques" 1–35 "be approved for use with unlawful combatants outside the United States" (Greenberg and Dratel 2005, 346–347).

6. A public secret is one shared by the majority of people but never publicly acknowledged. See Michael Taussig (1999) for further discussion.
7. See chapter 5 of *Political Bodies/Body Politic: The Semiotics of Gender* (Juschka 2009) for a discussion of masculinity and war.
8. For a reading of the Marquis de Sade and the link between sexuality, power and pain see Carter (1990).
9. For a developed discussion of race and masculinity see Kimmel and Messner (2007).
10. According to the 2007 US Census 51% of US citizens consider themselves to be Protestant (Pew Forum 2008), while currently that number appears to have dropped to 43%, according to a report from Pew Research Center (2019).
11. I follow Thomas Laqueur (1992), who argues that from 1800 onward, the male and female are conceptualized as opposite sexes and genders in the Eurowest.
12. According to Mark Kermode in his 2004 review of the film, "Crucial to the movie's success in America has been the mobilization of Christian groups who have block-booked screenings for their followers and orchestrated widespread congregational support. In Dallas, Christian businessman Arch Bonnema reserved an entire 20-screen cinema to play *The Passion* to more than 6,000 viewers on its opening day" (Kermode 2004). Roger Ebert commented in his review that "[t]he movie is 126 minutes long, and I would guess that at least 100 of those minutes, maybe more, are concerned specifically and graphically with the details of the torture and death of Jesus. This is the most violent film I have ever seen" (Ebert 2004).
13. Both these terms are derived from language adopted by US interrogators (see Jaffer and Singh 2007).
14. According to Jane Mayer, writing in the *New Yorker*, "the New Paradigm … rests on a reading of the Constitution that few legal scholars share namely, that the President, as Commander-in-Chief, has the authority to disregard virtually all previously known legal boundaries, if national security demands it. Under this framework, statutes prohibiting torture, secret detention, and warrantless surveillance have been set aside" (Mayer 2006).
15. See also Wisnewski (2010) and Rejali (2007) for a debunking of the effectiveness of torture for securing information or the "truth."
16. "Pride up and ego down" comes from the Army Field Manual and refers to "attacking the source's sense of personal worth," while "futility" refers to "making the source believe that it is useless to resist" (in Jaffer and Singh 2007, 9).
17. Page DuBois comments that in classical Athenian legal system, evidence from a slave could only be received if acquired through torture since the slave, due to his/her servile status, could not be trusted to speak the truth (DuBois 1991, 35–36). During the witchcraft and sorcery trials of the early modern period of France there were, "cultural beliefs that supported the practice of torture—that the truth was embodied and that pain might free it from its carnal location" (Silverman 2001, 83). Something akin to this operates in the logic of the ritual of torture-truth.

18. Rumsfeld famously wrote "I stand for 8–10 hrs a day. Why is standing limited to 4 hours?" on the bottom of the November 27, 2002 memo requesting permission to use this and other techniques of torture (for a copy of the memo see Greenberg and Dratel 2005, 236).

Chapter 5

1. Textualization is a process of abstraction even as it locates the words and gestures of orality in time and space. The linguistic double play of absence and presence is a primary site for ideological production (see Althusser 1995).
2. For discussions on the magical cures and ills of circumcision see Gollaher (2000), Henerey (2004), Kimmel (2001), Lyons (2013), Sarajlic (2014), Scolnic (2013), and Zabus (2008).
3. The *chicotte* is a braided whip developed specifically to apply to the black African, slave or force laborers, during this period by Belgium authorities. The whip and its application to the bodies of Indigenous people signified Eurowestern dominance: white, masculine, and capitalist (see Montineau 2018).
4. This view continues well into the present as Linda Villarosa so cogently demonstrates in her article "How False Beliefs in Physical Racial Difference Still Live in Medicine Today." She notes that: "A 2016 survey of 222 white medical students and residents published in The Proceedings of the National Academy of Sciences showed that half of them endorsed at least one myth about physiological differences between black people and white people, including that black people's nerve endings are less sensitive than white people's" (Villarosa 2019).
5. Acts served as foundational toward defining and determining Christianities in the second and third centuries (Arnal 2011, 202 ff.; Arnal 2008, 75 ff.).
6. Arnal (2011, 205) notes that the innovation of bringing together Acts and the Pauline letters allowed for the expansion of the heroic figuring of "Paul."
7. I want to thank William Arnal for the terms and their translation.
8. The term "suffering" finds its way into the Pauline letters, but it is really only one case, Romans 8:17, where bodily pain is meant rather than "not putting up with" something, although the latter meaning may be intended as well.
9. Prolificness refers to the commandment to be fruitful and multiple, something Philo took the foreskin to hamper.
10. Philo contends that circumcision is not required for humans marked as female/feminine as the *materia* or feminine cause was inert matter and therefore did not shape the nature of the child, while the feminine was not subject to "venereal pleasures" as much as the male (Philo 1993a, QG: 47).
11. Howard Eilberg-Schwartz argues that the Pauline texts' development of circumcision de-emphasizes Abrahamic genealogy and laid the ground for the myth of the human virgin-deity conception and birth of the semi-divine figure who then achieves full divinity upon death and apotheosis (Eilberg-Schwartz 1994, 229).

12. The writings of Philo intersect with the Abrahamic narrative reading circumcision as an outward sign of purity that is also meant to represents an inward state of purity: that is, the cut references a cutting away of the superfluous and excessive flesh of the foreskin that then references the cutting away of superfluous and excessive desires of the heart (Philo 1993a, 46).
13. Certainly there are variant versions of Genesis, but the necessity for circumcision on the eighth day remains consistent (Thiessen 2011, 18–30).
14. The text is also suggestive of a marriage rite, something circumcision was associated with among the peoples in the Levant such as at Ugarit (Wyatt 2009, 423–424).
15. Margaret Talbot's feminist rereading of Exodus 4:24-26 reintroduces pain to the text refocusing as she does on the unnamed child and the child's mother (Talbot 2017, 212–217). Like Mieke Bal (1988), who alerts the reader to the erasure of the subjectivity, pain, and murder of the concubine in the story of the Levite and the Concubine found in Judges 19, Talbot reorients the reader's view from an androcentric reading to one that treats Tsipporah and her son as meaningful to the narrative, regardless that Tsipporah and the unnamed child fall away from the Moses myth in Exodus 4:24.
16. For a discussion on war as male sacrifice see Juschka (2009, ch. 3).
17. Similar to the narrative of the mass circumcision and slaughter of the men of Shechem is the mythic narrative of Saul's bride price of one hundred Philistine foreskins for his daughter Michal in 1 Samuel. In the myth it was David who took up Saul's request and provided the foreskins of the Philistine warriors (1 Sam. 18:25-27). The foreskins acted to establish a relationship between Saul and David, and briefly deflected the murderous wrath of Saul; much as Tsipporah deflected the wrath of deity when she provided him with the foreskin and blood of her son.
18. Spell 17 indicates that Re gave birth to Hu and Sia from the drops of blood from his self-circumcision (Megahed and Vymazalova 2011, 158).

References

Agamben, Giorgio. 1998. *Homo Sacer. Sovereign Power and Bare Life*. Translated by Daniel Heller-Roazen. Stanford, CA: Stanford University Press.
Agamben, Giorgio. 2004. *The Open: Man and Animal*. Stanford, CA: Stanford University Press.
Althusser, Louis. 1971. *Lenin and Philosophy and Other Essays*. Translated by Ben Brewster. New York: Monthly Review Press.
Althusser, Louis. 1995. "Ideology and Ideological State Apparatuses (Notes Toward an Investigation)." In *Mapping Ideology*, ed. Slavoj Žižek, 100–140. London: Verso.
Anderson, B. 2006. *Imagined Communities: Reflections on the Origin and Spread of Nationalism*. Revised edition. New York: Verso.
Apollodorus. 1961–63. *The Library*. Translated by James George Fraser. Loeb Classical Library. Cambridge, MA: Harvard University Press; W. Heinemann.
Apuleius. 2011. *The Golden Ass*. Translated by Sarah Ruden. New Haven, CT: Yale University Press.
Aristophanes. 2000. *Birds, Lysistrata, Women at the Thesmophoria*. Edited and translated by Jeffrey Henderson. Loeb Classical Library. Cambridge, MA: Harvard University Press. https://doi.org/10.4159/dlcl.aristophanes-women_thesmophoria.2000
Aristotle. 1979. *Aristotle: Generation of Animals*. Loeb Classical Library No. 366. Translated by A. L. Peck. Cambridge, MA: Harvard University Press. https://doi.org/10.4159/dlcl.aristotle-generation_animals.1942
Arnal, William. 2011. "The Collection and Synthesis of 'Tradition' and the Second-Century Invention of Christianity." *Method and Theory in the Study of Religion* 23, no. 3–4: 193–215. https://doi.org/10.1163/157006811x608359
Arnal, William. 2008. "Doxa, Heresy, and Self-Construction: The Pauline Ekklesiai." In *Heresy and Identity in Late Antiquity*, eds. Edward Iricinschi and Holger Zellentin, 50–101. Tubingen, Germany: Mohr Siebeck. https://doi.org/10.4000/assr.21587
Bailey, E. I. 1997. *Implicit Religion in Contemporary Society*. Kampen, Netherlands: Kok Pharos.
Baker, Steve. 1993. *Picturing the Beast: Animals, Identity, and Representation*. Manchester: Manchester University Press.
Bal, Mieke. 1988. *Death & Dissymmetry: The Politics of Coherence in the Book of Judges*. Chicago Studies in the History of Judaism. Chicago, IL: University of Chicago Press
Bataille, Georges. 1989. *The Tears of Eros*. Translated by P. Connor. San Francisco, CA: City Lights Books.

Beekes, Robert. 2009. *Etymological Dictionary of Greek*. Indo-European Etymological Dictionary Series. Leiden: Brill. https://doi.org/10.1108/09504121011091114

Blank, S., et al. 2012. "Male Circumcision: Task Force on Male Circumcision." *Pediatrics* 130, no. 3 (September): 756–785. https://doi.org/10.1542/peds.2012-1990

Bloch, Maurice. 1986. *From Blessing to Violence: History and Ideology in Circumcision Ritual of the Merina of Madagascar*. Cambridge: Cambridge University Press. https://doi.org/10.1163/157006690x00277

Boardman, John. 1963. "Artemis-Orthia and Chronology." *The Annual of the British School at Athens* 58: 1–7. https://doi.org/10.1017/s0068245400013721

Bordo, Susan. 1993. *Unbearable Weight: Feminism, Western Culture, and the Body*. Berkeley, CA: University of California Press.

Bordo, Susan. 1999. *The Male Body: A New Look at Men in Public and in Private*. New York: Farrar, Straus and Giroux.

Bordo, Susan R., and Alison M. Jaggar, eds. 1989. *Gender/Body/Knowledge: Feminist Reconstructions of Being and Knowing*. New Brunswick, NJ: Rutgers University Press.

Bosanquet, R. C., Alan J. B. Wace, Guy Dickins, R. M. Dawkins, H. J. W. Tillyard, and Ramsay Traquair. 1906. *Laconia: II. Excavations at Sparta*. The Annual of the British School at Athens. Athens: British School at Athens. https://doi.org/10.1017/s0068245400008224

Boswell, John Eastburn. 1984. "Expositio and Oblatio: The Abandonment of Children and the Ancient and Medieval Family." *The American Historical Review* 89, no. 1: 10–33. https://doi.org/10.2307/1855916

Bourdieu, P. 2001. *Masculine Domination*. Translated by R. Nice. Stanford, CA: Stanford University Press.

Boyarin, Daniel. 1992. "This We Know to Be the 'Carnal Israel': Circumcision and the Erotic Life of God and Israel." *Critical Inquiry* 18, no. 3: 474–505. https://doi.org/10.1086/448642

Boyle, Gregory J., Ronald J Goldman, Steven Svoboda, and Ephrem Fernandez. 2002. "Male Circumcision: Pain, Trauma and Psychosexual Sequelae." *Journal of Health Psychology* 7, no. 2: 329–343. https://doi.org/10.1177/1359105302007000310

Brown, Peter. 1988. *The Body and Society: Men, Women, and Sexual Renunciation in Early Christianity*. Lectures on the History of Religions, no. 13. New York: Columbia University Press.

Brulotte, Eric L. 2002. "Artemis: Her Peloponnesian Abodes and Cults." In *Peloponnesian Sanctuaries and Cults*, edited by Robin Hagg, 179–182. Stockholm: Svenska Institutet i Athen.

Budin, Stephanie Lynn. 2016. *Artemis*. New York: Routledge.

Burstyn, Varda. 1999. *The Rites of Men: Manhood, Politics and the Culture of Sport*. Toronto: University of Toronto Press.

Butler, Judith. 1993. *Bodies That Matter: On the Discursive Limits of "Sex."* New York: Routledge.

Butler, Judith. 1999. *Gender Trouble: Feminism and the Subversion of Identity*. New York; London: Routledge.

Butler, Judith. 2003. "Performative Acts and Gender Constitution." In *The Feminism and Visual Culture Reader*, edited by A. Jones, 392-402. New York: Routledge.
Butler, Judith. 2004. *Undoing Gender*. New York: Routledge.
Campbell, David A., trans. 1982-93. *Greek Lyric*. The Loeb Classical Library, vol. 144, no. 461. Cambridge, MA: Harvard University Press.
Campbell, Greg. 2012. *Blood Diamonds: Tracing the Deadly Path of the World's Most Precious Stones*. Revised edition. New York: Basic Books.
Campbell, Kirsten. 2004. *Jacques Lacan and Feminist Epistemology*. New York: Routledge.
Carr, David M. 2011. *The Formation of the Hebrew Bible: A New Reconstruction*. New York: Oxford University Press.
Carter, A. 1990. *The Sadeian Woman: An Exercise in Cultural History*. London: Virago.
Carter, Jane B. 1986. "Masks and Poetry in Early Sparta." In *Early Greek Cult Practice*. Proceedings of the Fifth International Symposium at the Swedish Institute at Athens, edited by Robin Hagg, Nanno Marinatos, and Gullog Nordquist, 89-104. Stockholm: Skrifter Utgivna av Svenska Institutet I Athens. https://doi.org/10.1017/s0003598x0007530x
Carter, Jane B. 1987. "The Masks of Ortheia." *American Journal of Archaeology* 19, no. 3 (July): 355-383.
Cartledge, Paul. 2001. *Spartan Reflections*. Berkeley, CA: University of California Press.
Cartledge, Paul. 2007. *Thermopylae: The Battle That Changed the World*. New York: Vintage Books.
Centers for Disease Control and Prevention. 2018. *HIV Surveillance Report, 2017*. Atlanta, GA: Centers for Disease Control and Prevention.
Chandler, Daniel. 2007. *Semiotics: The Basics*. 2002. New York: Routledge.
Chodorow, Nancy J. 1978. *The Reproduction of Mothering: Psychoanalysis and the Sociology of Gender*. Berkeley, CA: University of California Pres.
Christenson, Allen J., trans. 2004. *Popol Vuh Volume II: Literal Poetic Version, Translation and Transcription*. New York: O Books.
Christenson, Allen J., trans. and commentary. 2007. *Popol Vuh: Sacred Book of the Maya*. 2003. Norman, OK: University of Oklahoma Press.
Christien, Jacqueline. 2006. "The Lacadomanian State: Fortifications, Frontiers and Historical Problems." In *Sparta and War*, edited by Stephen Hodkinson and Anton Powell, 163-184. Swansea: Classical Press of Wales. https://doi.org/10.2307/j.ctvvnb23.8
Coakley, Sarah, ed. 1997. *Religion and the Body*. Cambridge Studies in Religious Traditions. Cambridge; New York: Cambridge University Press.
Coakley, Sarah. 2007. Introduction. In *Pain and Its Transformations: The Interface of Biology and Culture*, edited by Sarah Coakley and Kay Kaufman Shelemay, 1-16. Cambridge, MA: Harvard University Press. https://doi.org/10.1111/j.1748-0922.2009.01315_1.x
Coakley, Sarah, and Kay Kaufman Shelemay, eds. 2007. *Pain and Its Transformations: The Interface of Biology and Culture*. Cambridge, MA: Harvard University Press.
Coe, Michael. 1999. *The Maya*. 6th edition. London: Thames and Hudson.

Cooey, Paula M. 1994. *Religious Imagination and the Body: A Feminist Analysis.* New York: Oxford University Press.

Coogan, Michael, ed. 2001. *The New Oxford Annotated Bible: New Revised Standard Version with the Apocyrpha.* Oxford: Oxford University Press.

Cooper, David, Alex Wodak, and Brian Morris. 2010. "The Case for Boosting Infant Male Circumcision in the Face of Rising Heterosexual Transmission of HIV." *Medical Journal of Australia* 193, no. 6: 318–319. https://doi.org/10.5694/j.1326-5377.2010.tb03940.x

Cowan, John. 1970. *The Science of a New Life.* 1897. New York: Source Book Press.

Daly, Mary. 1978. *Gynecology: The Metaethics of Radical Feminism.* Boston, MA: Beacon Press.

Danforth, Loring. 1989. *Firewalking and Religious Healing: The Anastenaria of Greece and the American Firewalking Movement.* Princeton, NJ: Princeton University Press.

Darby, Robert. 2013. "The Child's Right to an Open Future: Is the Principle Applicable to Non-Therapeutic Circumcision?" *Journal of Medical Ethics* 39, no. 7 (January 1930): 463–468. https://doi.org/10.1136/medethics-2012-101182

Darby, Robert, and Laurence Cox. 2008. "Objections of a Sentimental Character: The Subjective Dimensions of Foreskin Loss." In *Fearful Symmetries Essays and Testimonies around Excision and Circumcision*, edited by Chantal J. Zabus, 145–168. Amsterdam: Editions Rodopi. https://doi.org/10.1163/9789042030619_007

Darby, Robert, and Robert Van Howe. 2011. "Not a Surgical Vaccine: There Is No Case for Boosting Infant Male Circumcision to Combat Heterosexual Transmission of HIV in Australia." *Australian and New Zealand Journal of Public Health* 35, no. 5: 459–465. https://doi.org/10.1111/j.1753-6405.2011.00761.x

Darwin, Charles. 1963. *The Origin of Species: By Means of Natural Selection of the Preservation of Favoured Races in the Struggle for Life.* Edited by Hampton L. Carson. New York: Washington Square Press.

Darwin, Charles. 1981. *The Descent of Man and Selection in Relation to Sex.* With an introduction by John Tyler Bonner and Robert M. May. Princeton, NJ: Princeton University Press.

Dave, S. S., K. A. Fenton, C. H. Mercer, B. Erens, K. Wellings, and A. M. Johnson. 2003. "Male Circumcision in Britain: Findings from a National Probability Sample Survey. Sexually Transmitted Infections." *Sexually Transmitted Infections* 79, no. 6 (December): 499–500. https://doi.org/10.1136/sti.79.6.499

Dawkins, Richard. 2004. *The Ancestor's Tale: A Pilgrimage to the Dawn of Evolution.* Boston, MA: Houghton Mifflin.

de Certeau, Michel. 1988. *The Writing of History.* Translated by Tom Conley. New York: Columbia University Press.

de Certeau, Michel. 1993. "History, Science and Fiction." In *History, Science and Fiction*, translated by Brian Massumi, 199–224. Minneapolis, MN: University of Minnesota Press.

Delaney, Carol. 1995. "Untangled the Meaning of Hair in Turkish Society." In *Off with Her Head: The Denial of Women's Identity in Myth, Religion, and Culture*, edited by

Howard Eilberg-Schwartz and Wendy Doniger, 53–75. Berkeley, CA: University of California Press. https://doi.org/10.2307/1399885

Descartes, René. 1924. *Discourse on the Method of Rightly Conducting the Reason, and the Seeking Truth in the Sciences.* Chicago, IL: The Open Court Publishing Company.

Douglas, Mary. 1966. *Purity and Danger: An Analysis of Concepts of Pollution and Taboo.* London: Penguin.

Douglas, Mary. 1970. *Natural Symbols: Explorations in Cosmology.* New York: Pantheon.

DuBois, Page. 1991. *Torture and Truth.* New York: Routledge.

Ducat, Jean. 2006a. *Spartan Education: Youth and Society in the Classical Period.* Swansea: Classical Press of Wales.

Ducat, Jean. 2006b. "The Spartan 'Tremblers'." In *Sparta and War*, edited by Stephen Hodkinson and Anton Powell, 1–56. Swansea: Classical Press of Wales. https://doi.org/10.2307/j.ctvvnb23.4

Ebert, R. 2004. "The Passion of the Christ." *Chicago Sun-Times*, February 24.

Eco, Umberto. 1979. *A Theory of Semiotics.* Bloomington, IN: Indiana University Press.

Eilberg-Schwartz, Howard. 1990. *The Savage in Judaism: An Anthropology of Israelite Religion and Ancient Judaism.* Bloomington, IN: Indiana University Press.

Eilberg-Schwartz, Howard. 1994. *God's Phallus and Other Problems for Men and Monotheism.* Boston, MA: Beacon Press.

Enloe, C. 2004. *The Curious Feminist: Searching for Women in the New Age of Empire.* Berkeley, CA: University of California Press.

Euripides. 1938. "Iphigenia in Tauris." Translated by Robert Potter. In *The Complete Greek Drama*, edited by Whitney J. Oates and Eugene Jr O'Neill, Jr. New York: Random House.

Foucault, Michel. 1972. *The Archaeology of Knowledge and the Discourse on Language.* Translated by A. M. Sheridan Smith. New York: Harper & Row.

Foucault, Michel. 1973. *The Order of Things: An Archaeology of the Human Sciences.* New York: Vintage.

Foucault, Michel. 1978. *An Introduction.* Vol. 1, *The History of Sexuality.* Translated by Robert Hurley. New York: Vintage.

Foucault, Michel. 1979. *Discipline and Punishment: The Birth of the Prison.* Translated by A. Sheridan. New York: Vintage.

Foucault, Michel. 1980a. *An Introduction.* Vol. 1, *The History of Sexuality.* Translated by Robert Hurley. New York: Vintage.

Foucault, Michel. 1980b. *Power/Knowledge: Selected Writings and Other Interviews 1972-1977.* Edited by Colin Gordon. Translated by Colin Gordon, Leo Marshal, John Mepham, and Kate Soper. New York: Pantheon.

Foucault, Michel. 1984. "Nietzsche, Genealogy, History." In *The Foucault Reader*, edited by Paul Rabinow, 76–100. New York: Pantheon Books.

Fowler, Robert. 2004. "The Homeric Question." In *The Cambridge Companion to Homer*, edited by Robert Fowler, 220–232. Cambridge: Cambridge University Press. https://doi.org/10.1017/ccol0521813026.014

Freud, Sigmund. 2005. *The Unconscious.* Translated by Graham Frankland. New York: Penguin Classics.
Gaca, Kathy L. 2015. "Ancient Warfare and the Ravaging Martial Rape of Girls and Women: Evidence from Homeric Epic and Greek Drama." In *Sex in Antiquity: Exploring Gender and Sexuality in the Ancient World*, edited by Mark Masterson, Nancy Sorkin Rabinowitz, and James Robson, 278–297. New York: Routledge. https://doi.org/10.33776/ec.v20i0.2949
Garenne M. 2008. "Long-Term Population Effect of Male Circumcision in Generalised HIV Epidemics in Sub-Saharan Africa." *African Journal of AIDS Research* 7, no. 1: 1–8. https://doi.org/10.2989/ajar.2008.7.1.1.429
Glucklich, Ariel. 2001. *Sacred Pain: Hurting the Body for the Sake of the Soul.* Oxford: Oxford University Press.
Goldenberg, Naomi R. 1993. *Resurrecting the Body: Feminism, Religion and Psychotherapy.* New York: Crossroad.
Gollaher, David. 2000. *Circumcision: A History of the World's Most Controversial Surgery.* New York: Basic Books.
Graf, Fritz. 2009. *Apollo.* New York: Routledge.
Greenberg, K. J., and J. L. Dratel, eds. 2005. *The Torture Papers: The Road to Abu Ghraib.* Introduction by A. Lewis. New York: Cambridge University Press.
Grosz, Elizabeth A. 1990. *Jacques Lacan: A Feminist Introduction.* London: Routledge.
Grosz, Elizabeth A. 1994. *Volatile Bodies: Toward a Corporeal Feminism.* Bloomington, IN: Indiana University Press.
Grosz, Elizabeth A. 1995. *Space, Time, and Perversion: Essays on the Politics of Bodies.* New York: Routledge.
Guerrini, Anita. 1989. "The Ethics of Animal Experimentation in Seventeenth-Century England." *Journal of the History of Ideas* 50, no. 3 (July–September): 391–407. https://doi.org/10.2307/2709568
Haddad, N, JS Li, S Totten, and M McGuire. 2018. *HIV in Canada-Surveillance Report, 2017.* Ottawa: Can Commun Dis Rep.
Hall, Stuart, ed. 1997. *Representation: Cultural Representations and Signifying Practices.* Thousand Oaks, CA: Sage.
Hall, Stuart. 2000. "Question of Cultural Identity." In *Modernity: An Introduction to Modern Societies*, edited by Stuart Hall, David Held, Don Hubert, and Kenneth Thompson, 595–634. Malden, MA: Blackwell.
Haraway, Donna. 2003. *The Companion Species Manifesto: Dogs, People, and Significant Otherness.* Chicago, IL: Prickly Paradigm Press.
Haraway, Donna. 2008. *When Species Meet.* Minneapolis, MN: University of Minnesota Press.
Harding, Sandra, ed. 2004. *The Feminist Standpoint Theory Reader: Intellectual and Political Controversies.* New York: Routledge.
Hartsock, Nancy C.M. 1998. *The Feminist Standpoint Revisited and Other Essays.* Boulder, CO: Westview Press.

Heath, John. 2005. *The Talking Greeks: Speech, Animals, and the Other in Homer, Aeschylus, and Plato*. Cambridge: Cambridge University Press.
Henerey, Adam. 2004. "Evolution of Male Circumcision as Normative Control." *The Journal of Men's Studies* 12, no. 3: 265–276. https://doi.org/10.3149/jms.1203.265
Herdt, Gilbert. 1994. *Guardians of the Flutes: Idioms of Masculinity*. Chicago, IL: University of Chicago Press.
Herodotus. 1926. *Herodotus The Persian Wars Book 7*. Translated by A. D. Godley. Cambridge, MA: Harvard University Press.
Hochschild, Adam. 1998. *King Leopold's Ghost: A Story of Greed, Terror, and Heroism in Colonial Africa*. Boston, MA: Houghton Mifflin.
Hodkinson, Stephen, and Anton Powell, eds. 2006. *Sparta and War*. Swansea: Classical Press of Wales.
Homer. 1998. *The Odyssey*. Translated by A. T. Murray, revised by George Dimock. Loeb Classical Library. Cambridge, MA: Harvard University Press.
Homer. 1999. *The Iliad*. Translated by A. T. Murray, revised by William F. Wyatt. Loeb Classical Library. Cambridge, MA: Harvard University Press.
hooks, bell. 1992. *Black Looks: Race and Representation*. Boston, MA: South End Press.
Ingold, Tim, ed. 1988. *What is an Animal?* London: Unwin Hyman.
Ingold, Tim. 2000. *The Perception of the Environment: Essays on Livelihood, Dwelling and Skill*. New York: Routledge.
Irigaray, Luce. 1993. *Je, Tu, Nous. English*. Translated by Alison Martin. New York: Routledge.
Jacobs, Andrew S. 2012. *Christ Circumcised: A Study in Early Christian History and Difference*. Philadelphia, PA: University of Pennsylvania Press.
Jaffer, Jameel, and Amrit Singh. 2007. *Administration of Torture: A Documentary Record from Washington to Abu Ghraib and Beyond*. New York: Columbia University Press.
Josephus. 1895. *The Works of Flavius Josephus*. Buffalo, NY: John E. Beardsley.
Joyce, Rosemary. 2000. *Gender and Power in Prehispanic Mesoamerica*. Austin, TX: University of Texas press.
Juschka, Darlene. 2009. *Political Bodies/Body Politic: The Semiotics of Gender*. Sheffield: Equinox.
Juschka, Darlene. 2017. "Indigenous Women, Reproductive Justice and Indigenous Feminisms: A Narrative." In *Listening to the Beat of Our Drum: Indigenous Parenting in a Contemporary Society*, edited by Carrie Bourassa, Betty McKenna, and Darlene Juschka. Toronto: Demeter.
Juschka, Darlene. 2021. "The Construction of Gender in Ritual and Myth." In *A Companion to Gender History*, edited by Teresa Meade and Merry Wiesner-Hanks. 2nd edition 59–74. Hoboken, NJ: Wiley.
Kacker, Seema, Kevin Frick, Charlotte Gaydos, and Aaron Tobian. 2012. "Costs and Effectiveness of Neonatal Male Circumcision." *Archives of Pediatrics & Adolescent Medicine* 166, no. 10: 910–918. https://doi.org/10.1001/archpediatrics.2012.1440
Kalof, Linda. 2007. *Looking at Animals in Human History*. London: Reaktion Books.

Kermode, M. 2004. "Drenched in the Blood of Christ." *The Observer*, February 29.
Kimmel, Michael S. 2001. "The Kindest Un-Cut. (Jewish Parents Who Don't Circumcise Their Sons)." *Tikkun* 16, no. 3: 43–48.
Kimmel, M. S., and M. A. Messner, eds. 2007. *Men's Lives*. 7th edition. Toronto: Pearson.
Kleinman, Arthur, Veena Das, and Margaret Lock, eds. 1997. *Social Suffering*. Berkeley, CA: University of California Press.
Kristeva, Julia. 1982. *Pouvoirs de l'Horreur. English*. Translated by Leon S. Roudiez. New York: Columbia University Press.
Kristeva, Julia. 1987. *Tales of Love*. Translated by Leon S. Roudiez. New York: Columbia University Press
Kron, Uta. 1998. "Sickles in Greek Sanctuaries: Votive and Cultic Instruments." In *Ancient Greek Cult Practice from the Archaeological Evidence*, Proceedings of the Fourth International Seminar on Ancient Greek Cults, organized by the Swedish Institute at Athens, October 22–24, 1993, edited by Robin Hagg, 187–215. Stockholm: Skrifter Utgivna av Svenska Institutet I Athens. https://doi.org/10.2307/507430
Lacan, Jacques. 1968. *The Language of the Self: The Function of Language in Psychoanalysis*. Translated by Anthony Wilden. New York: Dell.
Lacan, Jacques. 1977. *Séminaire de Jacques Lacan. v. 11. Les Quatre Concepts Fondamentaux de la Psychanalyse. English*. Edited by Jacques-Alain Miller. Translated from the French by Alain Sheridan. International Psycho-Analytical Library, no. 106. London: Hogarth Press.
Lacan, Jacques. 2007. *Écrits: The First Complete Edition in English*. Translated by Bruce Fink. New York: W. W. Norton & Company. https://doi.org/10.1007/978-3-476-05728-0_9225-1
Lakoff, George, and Mark Johnson. 1999. *Philosophy in the Flesh: The Embodied Mind and Its Challenge to Western Thought*. New York: Basic Books.
Laqueur, Thomas. 1992. *Making Sex: Body and Gender from the Greeks to Freud*. Cambridge, MA: Harvard University Press.
Levinas, Emmanuel. 1969. *Totality and Infinity: An Essay on Exteriority*. Translated by Alphonso Lingis. Pittsburgh, PA: Duquesne University Press.
Lévi-Strauss, Claude. 1963. *Structural Anthropology*. Edited by Claire Jacobson and Brooke Grundfest Scheipf. London: Allen Lane.
Liddell, Henry George, and Robert Scott. 1968. *A Greek-English Lexicon*. Oxford: Clarendon Press.
Lincoln, Bruce. 1981. *Emerging from the Chrysalis: Studies in Rituals of Women's Initiation*. Cambridge MA: Harvard University Press.
Lincoln, Bruce. 1986. *Myth, Cosmos, and Society: Indo-European Themes of Creation and Destruction*. Cambridge, MA: Harvard University Press.
Lincoln, Bruce. 1989. *Discourse and the Construction of Society: Comparative Studies of Myth, Ritual and Classification*. Oxford: Oxford University Press.
Livesey, Nina E. 2007. "Circumcision as a Malleable Symbol: Treatments of Circumcision in Phil, Paul and Justin Martry." Dissertation, Southern Methodist University, University Park, TX.

Locke, John. 1975. *An Essay Concerning Human Understanding*. Edited by Peter Nidditch. Oxford: Oxford University Press.
Loraux, Nicole. 1977. *La 'Bella Mort" Spartiate*. Strasbourg: Association pour l'étude de la civilisation romaine.
Lovejoy, Arthur O. 1960. *The Great Chain of Being: A Study of the History of an Idea*. New York: Harper and Row.
Low, Denise. 1992. "A Comparison of the English Translations of a Mayan Text, the Popol Vuh." *Studies in American Indian Literatures* 4, no. 2-3 (Summer/Fall): 15-34.
Lyons, Barry. 2013. "Male Infant Circumcision as a 'HIV Vaccine'." *Public Health Ethics* 6, no. 1: 90-103. https://doi.org/10.1093/phe/phs039
Mack, Arien, ed. 1999. *Humans and Other Animals*. 1995. Columbus: Ohio State University Press.
Mayer, J. 2006. "The Hidden Power: The Legal Mind behind the White House's War on Terror." *The New Yorker*, July 3.
McClintock, Anne. 1995. *Imperial Leather: Race, Gender, and Sexuality in the Colonial Contest*. New York: Routledge.
McLaren, Margaret A. 2002. *Feminism, Foucault, and Embodied Subjectivity*. SUNY Series in Contemporary Continental Philosophy. Albany, NY: State University of New York Press.
Megahed, Mohamed, and Hana Vymazalova. 2011. "Ancient Egyptian Royal Circumcision from the Pyramid Complex of Djedkare." *Anthropologie* 49, no. 2: 155-164.
Midgley, Mary. 1995. *Beast and Man: The Roots of Human Nature*. New York: Routledge.
Miller, Frank. 2006. *300*. Colors by Lynn Varley. Milwaukee, OR: Dark Horse Comics.
Mohanram, Radhika. 1999. *Black Body: Women, Colonialism, and Space*. Public Worlds, vol. 6. Minneapolis, MN: University of Minnesota Press.
Montineau, Ann-Charlotte. 2018. "Chicotte." In *International Law's Object*, edited by Jessie Hohmann and Daniel Joyce, 182-190. Oxford: Oxford University Press.
Morris, Errol, director. 2008. *Standard Operating Procedure*. Sony Pictures.
Murray, G. N. 2007. "Zack Snyder, Frank Miller and Herodotus: Three Takes on the 300 Spartans." *Akroterion* 52: 11-35. https://doi.org/10.7445/52-0-50
Nioloutsos, Konstantinos. 2013. "Reviving the Past: Cinematic History and Popular Memory in *The 300 Spartans*." *Classical World* 106, no. 2 (Winter): 261-283. https://doi.org/10.1353/clw.2013.0030
Nunn, John F. 1996. *Ancient Egyptian Medicine*. London: British Museum Press.
Ong, Aihwa, and Michael G. Peletz, eds. 1995. *Bewitching Women, Pious Men: Gender and Body Politics in Southeast Asia*. Berkeley, CA: University of California Press.
Ortner, Sherry. 1974. "Is Female to Male as Nature is to Culture?" In *Woman, Culture, Society*, edited by M.Z. Rosaldo and L. Lamphere, 67-88. Stanford, CA: Stanford University Press.
Ortner, Sherry. 1996. *Making Gender: The Politics and Erotics of Culture*. Boston, MA: Beacon Press.

Pausanias. 1918. *Pausanias Description of Greece*. Translated by W. H. S. Jones. Loeb Classical Library. London: W. Heinemann.

Peirce, Charles Sanders. 1986. "Letters to Lady Welby." In *Critical Theory since 1965*, 639–644. Tallahassee, FL: Florida State University Press.

Peirce, Charles Sanders. 1991. *Peirce on Signs: Writings on Semiotic*. Edited by James Hoopes. Chapel Hill, NC: University of North Carolina.

Petropoulos, J. C. B. 2011. *Kleos in a Minor Key: Homeric Education of a Little Prince*. Washington, DC: Center for Hellenic Studies, Trustees for Harvard University.

Pettersson, Michael. 1992. *Cults of Apollo at Sparta: The Hyakinthia, the Gymnopaidiai*. Stockholm: Paul Astroms forlag.

Pew Forum. 2008. *US Religious Landscape Survey*. Washington, DC: The Pew Forum on Religion & Public Life.

Pew Research Center. 2019. *In US, Decline of Christianity Continues at Rapid Pace*. Washington, DC: Pew Research Center.

Philo. 1993a. "Questions and Answers on Genesis III." In *The Works of Philo: Complete and Unabridged*. Translated by C. D. Yonge. Peabody, MA: Hendrickson Publishers.

Philo. 1993b. "The Special Laws, I." In *The Works of Philo: Complete and Unabridged*. Translatedby C.D. Yonge. Peabody, MA: Hendrickson Publishers.

Philo. 1993c. "The Special Laws, II." In *The Works of Philo: Complete and Unabridged*. Translatedby C.D. Yonge. Peabody, MA: Hendrickson Publishers.

Plato. 1967. *Laws*. Translated by R. G. Bury. Cambridge, MA: Harvard University Press.

Plutarch. 1931a. "Apophthegmata Laconica." In Plutarch, *Moralia*. Translated by Frank Cole Babbitt. Loeb Classical Library. Cambridge, MA: Harvard University Press.

Plutarch. 1931b. "Instituta Laconica." In Plutarch, *Moralia*. Translated by Frank Cole Babbitt. Loeb Classical Library. Cambridge, MA: Harvard University Press.

Plutarch. 2000a. "Agis." In *Lives: Agis and Cleomenes, Tiberius and Gaius Gracchus, Philopoemen and Glaminius*. Translated by Bernadotte Perrin. Loeb Classical Library. Cambridge, MA: Harvard University Press.

Plutarch. 2000b. "Cleomenes." In *Lives: Agis and Cleomenes, Tiberius and Gaius Gracchus, Philopoemen and Glaminius*. Translated by Bernadotte Perrin. Loeb Classical Library. Cambridge, MA: Harvard University Press.

Plutarch. 2004. "Agesilaus." In *Lives: Agesilaus and Pompey Pelopidas and Marcellus*. Translated by Bernadotte Perrin. Loeb Classical Library. Cambridge, MA: Harvard University Press.

Plutarch. 2005. "Lycurgus." In *Lives: Theseus and Romulus, Lycurgus and Numa, Solon and Publicola*. Translated by Bernadotte Perrin. Loeb Classical Library. Cambridge, MA: Harvard University Press.

Quirke, Stephen. 2015. *Exploring Religion in Ancient Egypt*. Blackwell Ancient Religions. Chichester: Wiley Blackwell.

Rehle, Thomas, Leigh Johnson, Timothy Hallett, Mary Mahy, Kim, Helen Odido, Dorina Onoya, Sean Jooste, Olive Shisana, Adrian Puren, Bharat Parekh, and John Stover. 2015. "Comparison of South African National HIV Incidence Estimates:

A Critical Appraisal of Different Methods." *PLoS ONE* 10, no. 7: 1–5. https://doi.org/10.1371/journal.pone.0133255

Rejali, Darius. 2007. *Torture and Democracy*. Princeton, NJ: Princeton University Press.

Rios, K., and D. Mischkowski. 2019. Shaping Responses to Torture: What You Call It Matters. *Personality and Social Psychology Bulletin* 45, no. 6: 934–946. https://doi.org/10.1177/0146167218802830

Römer, Thomas. 2014. "Joshua's Encounter with the Commander of Yhwh's Army (Josh. 5:13-15): Literary Construction or Reflection of a Royal Ritual?" In *Warfare, Ritual, and Symbol in Biblical and Modern Contexts*, edited by Brad E. Kelle, Frank Ritchel Ames, and Jacob L Wright. Atlanta, GA: Society of Biblical Literature. https://doi.org/10.2307/j.ctt6wqb3g.7

Rosenberg, Jonah Lloyd. 2015. "The Masks of Orthia: Form, Function and the Origins of Theatre." *The Annual of the British School at Athens* 110: 247–261. https://doi.org/10.1017/s006824541500009x

Roth, Ann Macy. 1991. *Egyptian Phyles in the Old Kingdom: The Evolution of a System of Social Organization*. Studies in Ancient Oriental Civilization, no. 48. Chicago, IL: Oriental Institute of the University of Chicago.

Ruether, Rosemary Radford. 1985. *Women-Church: Theology and Practice of Feminist Liturgical Communities*. San Francisco, CA: Harper.

Ruether, Rosemary Radford. 1992. *Gaia*. San Francisco, CA: HarperSanFrancisco.

Rutherford, Richard. 1996. *Homer*. Oxford: Oxford University Press.

Sarajlic, Eldar. 2014. "Can Culture Justify Infant Circumcision?" *Res Publica: A Journal of Legal and Social Philosophy* 20, no. 4: 327–343. https://doi.org/10.1007/s11158-014-9254-x

Sauneron, Serge. 2000. *The Priests of Ancient Egypt*. With a foreword by Jean-Pierre Corteggiani, translated from the French by David Lorton. Ithaca, NY: Cornell University Press.

Scarry, Elaine. 1985. *The Body in Pain: The Making and Unmaking of the World*. New York: Oxford University Press.

Scherer, M., and M. Benjamin. 2006. "Other Government Agencies." Retrieved from www.salon.com/news/abu_ghraib/2006/03/14/chapter_5/print.html.

Scolnic, Benjamin Edidin. 2013. "Circumcision and Immortality." *Conservative Judaism* 64: 6–29. https://doi.org/10.1353/coj.2013.0037

Scott, Joan W. 1991. "The Evidence of Experience." *Critical Inquiry* 17, no. 4 (Summer): 773–797.

Scott, Joan W. 1992. "Experience." In *Feminists Theorize the Political*, edited by Judith Butler and Joan W. Scott, 22–40. New York: Routledge. https://doi.org/10.7202/1065247ar

Sebeok, Thomas A. 1991. *A Sign is Just a Sign*. Bloomington, IN: Indiana University Press.

Sebeok, Thomas A. 1994. *Signs: An Introduction to Semiotics*. Toronto: University of Toronto Press.

Sebeok, Thomas A. 2001. *Global Semiotics*. Bloomington, IN: Indiana University Press.

Seesengood, Robert Paul. 2010. *Paul: A Brief History*. Malden, MA: Wiley-Blackwell.

Sered, Susan Starr. 1994. *Priestess, Mother, Sacred Sister: Religions Dominated by Women.* New York: Oxford University Press.
Shell, Marc. 1997. "The Holy Foreskin; or Money, Relics and Judeo-Christianity." In *Jews and Other Differences: The New Jewish Cultural Studies*, edited by Jonathan Boyarin and Daniel Boyarin, 345–359. Minneapolis, MN: University of Minnesota Press.
Shisana, O, T. Rehle, L Simbayi, K. Zuma, S. Jooste, N Zungu, N. Labadarios, and Onoya D. 2014. *South African National HIV Prevalence, Incidence and Behaviour Survey, 2012.* Human Sciences Research Council. Cape Town: South Africa: HSRC Press.
Silverman, Eric K. 2004. "Anthropology and Circumcision." *Annual Review of Anthropology* 33: 419–445.
Silverman, Kaja. 1983. *The Subject of Semiotics.* New York: Oxford University Press.
Silverman, Kaja. 1992. *Male Subjectivity at the Margins.* New York: Routledge.
Silverman, Lisa. 2001. *Tortured Subjects: Pain, Truth, and the Body in Early Modern France.* Chicago, IL: Chicago University Press.
Sissa, Giulia, and Marcel Detienne. 2000. *Daily Life of the Greek Gods.* Translated by Janet Lloyd. Stanford, CA: Stanford University Press.
Smith, Jonathan Z. 1982. *Imagining Religion: From Babylon to Jonestown.* Chicago Studies in the History of Judaism. Chicago, IL: University of Chicago Press.
Snyder, Zack, director. 2007. *300.* Warner Brothers Pictures.
Sorokan, Todd S., Jane C. Finlay, and Ann L. Jefferies. 2015. "Newborn Male Circumcision." *Paediatrics Child Health* 20, no. 6: 311–315. https://doi.org/10.1093/pch/20.6.311
Spivak, Gayatri Chakravorty. 1987. *In Other Worlds: Essays in Cultural Politics.* New York: Methuen.
Stevenson, Robert Louis. 2004. *Strange Case of Dr. Jekyll and Mr. Hyde.* Edited by Richard Dury. Edinburgh: Edinburgh University Press.
Stewart, David. 2005. *The Incscriptions from Temple XIX at Palenque: A Commentary.* San Francisco, CA: Pre-Columbia Art Research Institute.
Stoler, A. L. 2002. *Carnal Knowledge and Imperial Power: Race and the Intimate in Colonial Rule.* Berkeley, CA: University of California Press.
Strathern, Marilyn. 1980. "No Nature, No Culture: The Hagen Case." In *Nature, Culture, Gender*, edited by Marilyn Strathern and Carol P. MacCormack, 174–223. Cambridge: Cambridge University Press. https://doi.org/10.1525/ae.1982.9.3.02a00200
Strathern, Marilyn, and Carol P. MacCormack, eds. 1980. *Nature, Culture, and Gender.* Cambridge: Cambridge University Press.
Talbot, Margaret Murray. 2017. "Tsipporah, Her Son and the Bridegroom of Blood: Attending to the Bodies in Ex. 4:24–26." *Religions* 8, no. 10: 205–220. https://doi.org/10.3390/rel8100205
Taussig, M. 1999. *Defacement: Public Secrecy and the Labor of the Negative.* Stanford, CA: Stanford University Press.
Tedlock, Dennis, ed. and trans. 1996. *Popol Vuh: The Definitive Edition of the Mayan Book of the Dawn of Life and the Glories of Gods and Kings.* New York: Touchstone.

Tedlock, Dennis. 2010. *2000 Years of Mayan Literature*. Berkeley, CA: University of California Press.
Thiessen, Matthew. 2011. *Contesting Conversion: Genealogy, Circumcision and Identity in Ancient Judaism and Christianity*. New York: Oxford University Press.
van Gennep, Arnold. 1960. *The Rites of Passage*. Translated by Monika B. Vizedom and Gabrielle L. Caffee, with an introduction by Solon T. Kimball. Chicago, IL: University of Chicago Press.
Van Howe, Robert. 2013. "Routine Infant Circumcision: Vital Issues That the Circumcision Proponents May Be Overlooking." In *Genital Cutting: Protecting Children from Medical, Cultural, and Religious Infringements*, edited by George Denniston, Frederick Hodges, and Marilyn Fayre Milos, 29–54. Dordrecht: Springer. https://doi.org/10.1007/978-94-007-6407-1_2
Van Howe, Robert S., and J. Steven Svoboda. 2008. "Neonatal Pain Relief and the Helsinki Declaration." *The Journal of Law, Medicine & Ethics* 36, no. 4: 803–823. https://doi.org/10.1111/j.1748-720x.2008.00339.x
Vernant, Jean-Pierre. 1991. *Mortals and Immortals: Collected Essays*. Edited and translated by Froma I. Zeitlan. Princeton, NJ: University of Princeton Press.
Villarosa, Linda. 2019. "How False Beliefs in Physical Racial Difference Still Live in Medicine Today." *The New York Times Magazine*, August 14. Retrieved from www.nytimes.com/interactive/2019/08/14/magazine/racial-differences-doctors.html
Waldau, Paul, and Kimberley Patton, eds. 2006. *A Communion of Subjects: Animals in Religion, Science, and Ethics*. New York: Columbia University Press.
Walker Bynum, Caroline. 1991. *Fragmentation and Redemption: Essays on Gender and the Human Body in Medieval Religion*. New York: Zone Books.
Weber, M. 2001. *The Protestant Ethic and the Spirit of Capitalism*. Translated by S. Kalberg. London: Taylor and Francis.
Webster. 2000. "Human." In *Webster's Third New International Dictionary, Unabridged*. Retrieved from http://unabridged.merriam-webster.com
Weedon, Chris. 1999. *Feminism, Theory, and the Politics of Difference*. Oxford: Blackwell Publishers.
Weedon, Chris. 2001. *Feminist Practice and Poststructuralist Theory*. 2nd edition. Oxford: Blackwell Publishers.
Winquist, Charles. 1998. "Person." In *Critical Terms for Religious Studies*, edited by Victor C. Taylor, 225–238. Chicago, IL: University of Chicago Press.
Wisnewski, J. 2010. *Understanding Torture: Contemporary Ethical Debates*. Edinburgh: Edinburgh University Press.
Wolfe, Cary. 2003a. *Animal Rites: American Culture, the Discourse of Species, and Posthumanist Theory*. Chicago, IL: University of Chicago Press.
Wolfe, Cary, ed. 2003b. *Zoontologies: The Question of the Animal*. Minneapolis, MN: University of Minnesota Press.
World Health Organization. 2017. *Voluntary Medical Male Circumcision for HIV Prevention in 14 Priority Countries in Eastern and Southern Africa: Progress Brief*. Geneva: World Health Organization.

Wyatt, Nick. 2009. "Circumcision and Circumstance: Male Genital Mutilation in Ancient Israel and Ugarit." *Journal for the Study of the Old Testament* 33, no. 4: 405–431. https://doi.org/10.1177/0309089209105687

Xenophon. 1918. *Helenica*, vol 2. Translated by Carleton Brownson. Loeb Classical Library. Cambridge, MA: Harvard University Press.

Xenophon. 1968a. "Agesilaus." In *Xenophon: Scripta Minora*. Translated by E. C. Marchant. Loeb Classical Library. Cambridge, MA: Harvard University Press.

Xenophon. 1968b. "Constitution of the Lacadaemonians." In *Xenophon: Scripta Minora*. Translated by E. C. Marchant. Loeb Classical Library. Cambridge, MA: Harvard University Press.

Yelle, Robert. 2013. *Semiotics of Religion: Signs of the Sacred in History*. London: Bloomsbury.

Young, Iris Marion. 2005. *On Female Body Experience: "Throwing Like a Girl" and Other Essays*. Studies in Feminist Philosophy. New York: Oxford University Press.

Zabus, Chantal J., ed. 2008. *Fearful Symmetries Essays and Testimonies around Excision and Circumcision*. Amsterdam: Editions Rodopi.

Zampieri, Nicola, Emanuela Pianezzola, and Cecilia Zampieri. 2008. "Male Circumcision through the Ages: The Role of Tradition." *Acta Pædiatrica* 97, no. 9: 1305–1307. https://doi.org/10.1111/j.1651-2227.2008.00917.x

Zeitlin, Froma, I. ed. 1991. *Jean-Pierre Vernant Mortals and Immortals: Collected Essays*. Princeton, NJ: University of Princeton Press.

Zucconi, Laura. 2007. "Medicine and Religion in Ancient Egypt." *Religion Compass* 1, no. 1: 26–37. https://doi.org/10.1111/j.1749-8171.2006.00004.x

Index

Note: numbers containing *n* refer to notes.

Abraham 140–141, 144–145, 146, 150
Abu Ghraib 4, 106, 108–109, 116, 117–121
   deaths of detainees at 117–118,
      119–120
   female US soldiers at 117, 118,
      120–121
   feminization of detainees at 118,
      119–120
   indexable sign of pain at 118, 119,
      120, 121, 154
   and indexical sign of pain 4, 118, 119,
      120, 121, 122, 123
   rite of torture at 118–121
   SERE program at 111
   "softening up" procedures at 117,
      118–119, 120–121, 164*n*16, 165*n*19
   and voyeurism of media 109
Achaeans 42, 48, 50, 52, 53, 55, 159
Achilles 38, 40–41, 44, 45–46, 50, 51, 52
Actaeon 39–40
Aeneas 44, 46, 47
Africa, circumcision and HIV/AIDS
      control in 4, 127–131, 149
   and colonialism/slavery/racism 129,
      130–131, 152
   evidence critiqued 128–129, 130
   and pain 130–131, 152, 155
Agamben, Giorgio 37–38
Agamemnon 38, 48
Agesilaus 72, 74, 75–76, 92, 94, 95–96, 97
Agis 72, 74, 80, 101
agoge 3, 67, 68–69, 73–74, 75, 77–78, 79,
      92, 98
   and Artemis-Ortheia rites *see*
      Artemis-Ortheia, altar of
   and *diamastigosis* 69, 84
   and festivals of Apollo *see* Apollonian
      festivals
   girls in 77, 87
   and Krypteia 69, 83–84, 86, 87, 93
   pain/violence in 81, 82, 91, 94–95, 97
   and singing/dancing/performance
      81, 82, 98
   and theft/punishment 8, 74, 77, 80,
      83, 84, 87, 95, 97
al-Qaeda *see* torture and war on terror
al-Qahtani, Mohammed 117
Alcman 87
algos/algeo 43, 44
Althusser, Louis 28, 156*n*3
Amarynceus 46, 47
Amyklaion 81
animal experimentation 25, 26, 36, 131
animal exploitation/cruelty 36, 37
animals, non-human 2, 3, 29, 154, 156*n*1
   as failed act of creation 59, 60, 61, 64
   ontology of 59–60
   and pain 15, 25–26, 36–37, 50, 56,
      65–66, 131, 157*n*11
   sacrificial 40, 50–51, 52, 54, 56, 90, 94,
      97, 161*nn*28, 29
   as tools/possessions 51, 52, 54, 56, 59
   Umwelt of 6–7, 37
   see also specific animals
animal–human binary 9, 23, 30–38
   as basis for binary set 31–32, 36

and belief systems 34–37
and boundaries/borders 37, 38, 39, 55, 158*n*10
and creation myths 58–59
and fear of devolution to the "beast" 30
and foundation myths 158*n*4
and hierarchy of senses 33–34
in *Iliad/Odyssey* 37, 38–43, 50–51, 54
and kinship 2–3, 37, 38, 39–40
and otherness of animals 42–43
and pain 25–26, 37, 50–51, 56, 131
in *Popol Vuh* 37, 58–60, 64–65
and science 32–34, 36
as social construction 31
and soul 36
and speech 38, 39, 40–43, 59–60
and transformation myths 39–40, 158–159*n*11
anthropogonic myths 2–3, 23, 34, 36, 38, 57, 64–65, 158*n*8
Aphrodite 44, 45, 47, 56
Apollo 38, 44, 45, 48, 49, 52, 73, 90, 94, 98, 104, 163*n*8
Apollo Karneios 82, 89, 98
Apollo Pytheaus 82, 98
Apollodorus 39–40
Apollonian festivals 80–83, 98–99
    ball game at (*Spairomachiai*) 82, 99
    Gymnopaidiai 80, 82, 88, 98–99
    Hyakinthia 80, 81–82, 88, 97, 98
    Karneia *see* Karneia
    pursuit/race at 82, 83
archeology 68, 84–87, 100–101
Ares 44, 45, 47, 52, 56
Aristophanes 67
Aristotle 29, 33, 34, 36, 67, 84, 99
Arnaeus/Irus 55, 161*n*35
Arnal, William 135, 165*nn*6, 7
Artemis 39–40, 80, 90, 97, 98, 104
Artemis Kourotrophos 103
Artemis-Ortheia, altar of 3, 76, 84–87, 88, 94, 98–102, 103

archeology of 68, 84–87, 100–101
cheese theft ritual at 80, 83, 84, 87, 97, 98, 99, 101
competitions held at 86–87
flogging ritual at *see* flagellation ritual
girls' rites of passage at 87
masks of 85–86, 87, 100
sickles of 85, 86–87, 101
xoanon at 84, 99, 101, 102
Asad, Talal 8
Athena 42, 44, 52, 55, 90, 162*n*2
Auilix 62, 63, 64
austerity 73, 74, 79
Australia 128, 133, 134

baptism 135–136, 139, 150
Bataille, Georges 27
Belgian Congo 129, 131, 149
Bible 34, 36
    see also Exodus; Genesis; Joshua; Paul
binaries 10, 38, 104, 153, 155, 156*nn*2, 4, 157–158*n*2
    as social constructions 158*n*3
    see also animal-human binary
biopolitics/biopower 7, 14–15
Bloch, Maurice 127
boar hunting 47, 53, 54, 55, 161*n*34
body 7–18, 154, 155
    as absent referent 10
    abstracted through textualization 124
    as constructed/performed 15–16, 23
    and feminism 7–8
    and matter/materialization 14, 15
    and pain 7, 15–18, 28, 38, 124
    and postmodernism 9–10
    and poststructuralism 10–11, 14–15
    and power 14–15, 157*n*8
    and psychoanalytic theory 11–14
    and racism/othering 9, 130–131, 134
    and Real/Imaginary/Symbolic 11–13, 14, 15–16
    and religion 7, 8–9

and semiotics 23–24
and social systems 9
theories of 2, 6, 7–15
and torture *see* torture
and truth 14, 156n2
and unconscious 13–14
body/soul-mind binary 10, 13, 14, 155
Bordo, Susan 7
boundaries/borders 37, 38, 54, 55, 158n10
  kinship as *see* kinship
  in *Popol Vuh* 64–66
  speech as *see* speech
  and torture 120
Bourdieu, Pierre 111
Britain (UK) 132, 133
Brown, Peter 8
brutes 25–26, 157n12
Bush, George W. 107, 109, 114, 115, 116, 120
Butler, Judith 2, 7, 14, 15, 16, 24, 28, 113, 156n7
  and discourse analysis 29
Bybee, Jay 109, 114, 115–116
Bynum, Caroline Walker 8

Campbell, Greg 129
Campbell, Kirsten 13
Canada 130, 132, 149–150
capitalism 112–113, 122
Carr, David 141
Carter, Angela 117
Carter, Jane 85–86, 162n3
Cartledge, Paul 67, 81, 85
Catholicism 27, 30, 121, 134
Chandler, Daniel 18
cheese theft ritual 80, 83, 84, 87, 97, 98, 99, 101
Cheney, Dick 107, 109
children/infants 1, 11–12, 41, 71–72, 156n1
  see also infant circumcision
Christenson, Allen 57, 58, 60, 63, 161n38

Christianity 8, 24, 27, 124, 153, 155
  and animal-human binary 25, 32, 34–37
  and masculinity 112
  see also Catholicism; Jesus Christ; Paul; Protestantism
Circe myth 39, 40
circumcision 4–5, 26, 124–153, 160n24
  in ancient Egypt 146–149, 151, 152–153, 154–155
  and baptism 135–136, 139, 150
  and construction of masculinities 125
  contexts/outcomes of 124–125
  and deity 135–136, 137, 139–141, 142–143, 144, 145, 146, 150, 151
  as disease prevention 126, 127, 132, 137–138, 149, 152, 165n2
  and foreskin as feminine 124, 125, 127
  genealogy of 4, 125, 153, 166n11
  and HIV/AIDS *see* Africa, circumcision and HIV/AIDS control in
  and identity 124, 128, 135, 138–139, 150
  as indexical sign 5, 125–126, 139, 140, 142, 143, 144, 145, 147–148, 149, 150–151, 152, 153
  and infants *see* infant circumcision
  and Josephus 138–139, 150
  and masculinity 124, 125–126, 127, 136, 137, 143, 149, 150, 153
  and masturbation/desire 126, 132, 137, 138, 149–150, 152
  and pain 124, 125, 130–131, 133–134, 136–137, 140, 143, 145, 148, 149, 150, 151, 152, 153
  and Paul 34, 134–136, 138, 139, 149, 150
  and Philo 136–138, 139, 149, 150–151, 152
  and progress/social evolutionism 126–127

and purity 124, 125, 126, 127, 132, 137, 138, 139, 144, 148, 149, 152, 166n12
and reproduction 137, 140, 146, 151, 165n9
as sacrifice 13, 140, 142, 143–144, 145, 146, 151, 152, 154
and *Tanakh* 139–146, 149, 151–152, 166n17
and warfare 143–144, 145–146, 151–152
see also foreskin
class 2, 38, 112–113, 132
Cleomenes 72, 74–75
Coakley, Sarah 8, 17
colonialism 8, 25–26, 31, 126, 163n1
and circumcision 129, 131, 149, 152
and Mayans 56
Constantine 105
Constitution of the Lacedaemonians (Xenophon) 70, 76, 77, 78, 90, 97, 99
Cooper, David 128
Coronea, Battle of 75, 76
cosmogonic myths 2, 23, 60
Cowan, John 126–127
Cox, Laurence 134
Cranach, Lucas 27
creation myths 57–58
anthropogonic 2–3, 23, 34, 36, 38, 57, 64–65, 158n8
cosmogonic 2, 23, 60
demogonic 3, 38, 64–65, 158n8
Crusoe, Robinson 21–22
culture 8, 9, 13
and nature, binary of 23, 28, 32, 33, 36

Darby, Robert 128–129, 132–133, 134
Darwin, Charles 30, 33
Dave, S. S. 132
de Sade, Marquis 27, 117
deities

and animal-human binary 2, 3, 31, 39, 40, 41, 54, 56
and creation myths 57–60
and horses 52
pain inflicted by 104–105, 163n8
pain of 45, 47, 50, 54, 55–56, 60, 160n23
and rituals/sacrifice 26, 28, 62–63, 64
see also specific deities
demogonic myths 3, 38, 62, 64–65, 158n8
Descartes, René 25, 26, 33, 36–37, 131, 160n27
Deuteronomy 145
diamastigosis see flagellation ritual
Didacus Valades 34–36
Diomedes 44, 45, 46, 47, 48, 50, 55
discomposing 29–30
discourse analysis 29
dogs 36, 50, 53, 131, 155
hunting 40, 51
used in torture 116, 119
Dolon 50, 52, 54–55
Doniger, Wendy 8
Douglas, Mary 8
DuBois, Page 17, 24, 111, 164–165n18
Ducat, Jean 77, 78–79, 84, 86, 162n7
Dunlavey, Gen. Michael 109, 116

Eco, Umberto 18, 21, 22–23, 24, 157n9
Egypt 4, 73, 75, 76, 125, 126, 136
circumcision in 146–149, 151, 152–153, 154–155, 166n18
see also Exodus
Eilberg-Schwartz, Howard 139, 140, 141, 166n11
empiricism 1, 8
endurance of pain 47, 50, 74, 81, 82, 83, 88, 94, 97, 98, 99
England, Lynndie 120–121
Enlightenment 32, 131
Enloe, C. 113–114
ephebes 47, 48, 49, 86, 87

Ephialtes 69, 70
Ephors/ephorate 70, 74–75, 76, 78, 85, 88, 89, 92
epistemes 38, 158n7
epistemology 7, 9, 32, 110
eroticism 27, 121
Eurowest
    and animal-human binary 32–34
    and the body 7–8, 10, 15, 16, 17
    and circumcision 124, 130–131
    and pain 26
    and sexuality 29–30
    and terrorism 107
evolutionary theory 30, 33
Exodus 139–140, 141–143, 144, 145, 146, 149, 151, 152, 166n15
experience 154

father 12–13
female/feminine 9, 10, 74, 165n10
    foreskin as 124, 125, 127
    heroic 71
    of Islamic other 4, 106, 120, 154
    and masculine, binary of 31, 49, 155, 157–158n2, 164n11
    and penetration 111
    and terrorism 107
feminism 6, 166n15
    and the body 7, 9
    postmodern 9–10
    poststructural 1, 2, 7
fire-walking 104–105
flagellation ritual 69, 76, 84, 87, 95, 101–102, 103, 155
    and *xoanon* 99, 101, 102
foreskin
    as feminine 124, 125, 127
    as impure 124, 125, 126, 127, 132, 137, 138, 149
    of Jesus 127–128
    and magical power 127
Foucault, Michel 2, 7, 65, 124, 157n8, 158n7

and discourse analysis 29–30
    on power 10, 14–15, 107
fourmother-fathers 58, 59, 62, 63, 64
Fowler, Robert 38
France 107, 117, 163n2, 165n18
freedom 70, 88–89, 92, 93
Freud, Sigmund 11, 13–14, 33–34, 156nn5, 6

Gaca, Kathy 103
Galucus 48–49
Garenne, A. 128–129
Gaza, Israeli attacks on 107
gender 2, 29, 38, 101, 106
genealogy 27, 58, 124
    of circumcision 4, 125, 141, 153, 166n11
Genesis 34, 36, 139–141, 143–145, 146, 151, 166n13
gerousia 75, 89
Gibson, Mel 24, 27, 114
Goldenberg, Naomi 8
Gollaher, David 127, 129
Gonzales, Alberto 109, 114, 115
Gorgo 3–4, 70, 71, 162n2
Gorgon 71, 162n2
    masks 85–86, 100
Graner, Charles 120–121
great chain of being 34–36, 158n5
Greece 3, 72, 76, 80, 81, 82, 93, 103, 104–105
    see also Homeric texts; Spartan masculinity
Grosz, Elizabeth 2, 7, 11, 156n3
Guantánamo Bay 109, 116, 117, 163n2
Guatemala 56–57
Gymnopaidiai 80, 82, 88, 98–99, 162n7

Hacauitz 62, 63, 64
Hall, Stuart 17, 29
Harman, Sabrina 120–121
Heath, John 39, 41, 159nn13, 16, 160n18
Hector 38, 42–43, 49, 50

helots 72, 75–76, 95
  rite of hunting *see* Krypteia
Henerey, Adam 126, 132
Hera 38, 40, 44, 45, 52, 54, 87, 158n11
Heracles 76, 87, 94, 159n12
Herdt, Gilbert 17, 24, 26
Hermes 87, 159n11
Herodotus 71, 72, 79, 111, 146
heroic ethos 46, 47–48, 50, 56, 159n16, 161n32
  see also warrior masculinity
heroines 71
heteronormativity 88, 94
heterosexuality 29, 30, 111
  and HIV/AIDS 128, 129, 133
history 7, 9
HIV/AIDS 132–133, 149
  see also Africa, circumcision and HIV/AIDS control in
Hochschild, Adam 129, 131
Hodkinson, Stephen 70
Homeric texts 43–56, 73
  animal-human binary in 37, 39, 43, 65–66
  authoritative speech in 41
  pain in 43–46
  self in 49
  shrieking in 50, 54–55
  significations of pain in 54–56
  terms for pain in 43–44, 160nn19, 21
  warrior masculinity in 3
  wrath/rage in 45–46
  see also Iliad; Odyssey
homophobia 109
homosexuality 29, 112
hooks, bell 7
hoplites *see* Spartan masculinity
horses 51, 52–54
  and pain 50, 52, 53–54
humiliation 106, 110, 111, 116, 117, 118
Hunahpu 61–62, 64, 161n37
hunting 40, 47, 51, 53, 54, 103, 161n34
Hyakinthia 80, 81–82, 88, 98

Hyakinthos 81, 98, 104, 105
hybrid creatures 44, 159n12

icons 17, 19, 21, 22
  and body 23
ideology 14
Iliad 2, 31, 37, 38–39, 65
  horses in 52, 53, 56
  otherness of animals in 42–43
  pain in 43–47, 48–50
  pain in, terms for 43, 44, 160nn19, 21
  pain of animals in 50–52
  self in 49
  shrieking in 50, 54–55
  speech in 41–43
  transformation myths in 40–41, 158–159n11
  wrath/rage in 45–46
Imaginary order 11–12, 13, 15
indexical sign 18, 19–23
  and body 23
  and circumcision 125, 128
  and mode of secondness 21, 90
indexical sign of pain 2–3, 7, 18, 25, 28, 154–155
  and animal-human binary 37
  and boundaries 54, 55
  and circumcision/scarification 4–5, 26, 27, 125–126
  in Homeric texts 44, 49–50, 54, 55
  and performance 23
  in *Popol Vuh* 57, 60–61, 66
  and Spartan masculinity 67, 82, 87, 90–91, 94–95, 97, 99, 100, 102, 104
  as symbol 22
  and symptoms 21
  and torture 106, 110, 114
  and war on terror *see under* torture and war on terror
infant circumcision 125, 131–134, 147, 148, 152
  and class 132
  and pain 133–134, 136, 140

and proxy consent/rights in trust 133
and *Tanakh* 141, 144, 145, 146, 150, 166n13
and trauma in later life 134
Iolaos 87
Iphigenia 101, 102, 105, 163n8
Iraq, invasion of (2003) 113
  see also Abu Ghraib
Irigaray, Luc 7
Irus/Arnaeus 55, 161n35
Isaac 140, 141, 146, 154
Ishmael 140, 141
Islam 8, 34, 122, 124, 126
Islamic other 4, 106, 120, 154
Israel 107
Israelite warriors 140, 143–144, 145, 146, 151–152, 154–155
Izates of Parthian 138

Jackson, Peter 70
Jaffer, Jameel 111, 115–116, 117, 118, 119, 163nn2, 3, 164n17
Jagger, Allison 7
Jesus Christ 24, 27, 136, 150, 164n12
Johnson, Mark 28
Josephus 138–139, 150
Joshua 139–140, 143–144, 145, 146, 149, 151–152, 154
Judaism/Jews 8, 34
  and circumcision 124, 126, 128, 135, 136, 137–139

Kalof, Linda 131
Kant, Immanuel 37
Karneia 80, 82–83, 88, 98
  pursuit/race at 82, 83, 89
Kimmel, Michael 134
kinship 2–3, 37
  in Homeric texts 38, 39–40, 53, 160n18
  in *Popol Vuh* 57–59, 64, 65
Kipling, Rudyard 30, 149
knowledge systems 24, 37
  see also Umwelt

Kristeva, Julia 7
Kron, Uta 86–87
Krypteia 69, 83–84, 87, 88, 93, 99–100, 103, 104

laboring animals 52, 54, 56, 59
Lacan, Jacques 2, 7, 11–13, 14, 15, 156n1
Lakoff, George 28
language 1–2
  and body 9–11
  and masculinity 12
  as modelling device 10–11
  and pain 1–2, 6, 17–18, 24, 105
Laqueur, Thomas 29
Leonidas 3–4, 67, 68, 69, 71, 72, 79, 88, 89, 91, 104
Leto 46, 98
Lévi-Strauss, Claude 11, 157n13
Lewis, Anthony 114, 115
Liddell, Henry George 43, 44, 161n34
liminal space/liminality 81, 98, 103, 118, 119, 162n6
  and circumcision 135, 141
  and torture 109, 115
Lincoln, Bruce 26–27, 120, 157n14
Livesey, Nina 137
Locke, John 36–37, 157n11
Lord of the Rings, The (film) 70
Lycurgus 72–73, 79, 92, 93, 96, 97
  laws of 70, 73, 76, 77, 78, 94, 96, 101, 103

Mack, Arien 29
Madagascar 127
magic 22, 127
male/masculine 10, 12
  and authoritative speech 43
  and circumcision *see under* circumcision
  and feminine, binary of 31, 49, 155, 157–158n2, 164n11
  improper, sign of 52, 55, 66, 154, 155
  and pain 4, 25, 46, 47–48, 66

and penetration *see* penetration
and penis/phallus formation 125
racialized 112
and torture 110, 111, 120–121, 122
warrior *see* warrior masculinity
white US 106, 110–114
manikins 58, 59, 61, 63
masks 85–86, 87, 100
masturbation 30, 118, 126, 132, 149–150, 152
Maté, Rudolph 72
Mattathias 138
matter/materialiation 14, 15
Mayans 56
time-line of 161n36
see also Popol Vuh
media 109, 113, 114
medicine 30
Medusa 86, 87, 162n2
Megahed, Mohamed 147
Menelaus 42–43, 50, 105
Merina people 127
Messenia/Messenians 75–76, 83, 85, 93, 95, 99
metonymy 20, 32, 90, 156n4
Midgley, Mary 8, 158n10
Miller, Frank *see* 300 (film/graphic novel, 2007/1998)
Miller, Gen. Geoffrey 109, 114, 116
mind 39
see also body/soul-mind binary
Mohanram, Radhika 7
Moses 141–142, 143, 144, 145, 146, 150, 151
mother–child dyad 11, 12
Mowhoush, Abed Hamed 119
mules 45, 50, 51–52
Murray, A. T. 44–45
Myanmar 65
myth 2, 3, 25, 28, 37–38, 158n4
transformation 39–40, 61, 158–159n11
see also creation myths
mythemes 26, 31, 70, 157n13

nature 15, 156n2
and culture, binary of 23, 28, 32, 33, 36
9/11 attacks 4, 106–107, 109, 121, 122

Odysseus 38, 40, 50, 52, 54–55
rite of passage of 47–48, 160n25
Odyssey 2, 37, 39, 40, 65
pain in 43, 44, 46, 47
shrieking in 54
status of horses/dogs in 52–53
terms for pain in 43, 44, 160nn19, 21
One Monkey/One Artisan 61
ontology 7, 34, 36, 38, 55, 59–60, 155
Orestes 101, 102, 105, 163n8
Ortheia 84, 85, 86
see also Artemis-Ortheia, altar of
othering/otherness 9, 65, 127, 133
and torture 106–107, 108, 109, 110, 113, 119, 120, 122
Ouranos 86, 87
oxen 50, 51

pain 15–18, 25–28
as constructed/performed 2, 16
of deities 44–45, 47
as external object 24, 28
as indexical sign *see* indexical sign of pain
and language 1–2, 6, 17–18, 25
and masculinity 4, 25, 46, 47–49
and masks 86
narratives of 17, 18
in *Popol Vuh* 60–64
and power 26
and racism 130–131, 134
and ritual 26–27
and self 49
semiotics of 19–20, 23–24, 25
and truth 17, 24, 25, 26, 28, 49, 91, 103, 154, 164n15, 164–165n19
visual discourse of 27, 49–50
Paris 42–43, 48, 49, 50

Passion of the Christ, The (film) 24, 27, 114, 164n12
Passover 143, 144, 151
Patroclus 44, 51, 53, 161n32
Paul 34, 134–136, 138, 139, 149, 150, 166n11
Pausanius 101–102
Pedasus (horse) 53, 54
Peirce, Charles Sanders 2, 7, 18–20, 22, 24, 90
penetration
 terrorism as 4, 106, 107, 122
 torture as 109, 110–112, 113, 115, 121, 122
penis/phallus formation 125, 126
performativity 16, 23
Persian army 3, 4, 67, 68, 69, 70, 71, 88–89
 as feminine 88, 104
Petropoulos, J. C. B. 47, 49, 160nn24, 25
Petterssen, Michael 80–81, 82, 83, 84, 86, 87, 89, 98, 99
phallus 125, 126
Philo 136–138, 139, 149, 150–151, 152, 166n12
Pianezzola, Emanuela 126
Plato 34, 67, 84, 99, 124
Plutarch 4, 7, 71, 72–76, 79–80, 88, 92–95, 96
 on Agesilaus 72, 74, 75–76, 92
 on Agis 72, 74, 80
 on Cleomenes 72, 74–75
 on flagellation ritual 76, 84, 87, 99, 101, 103
 and indexical sign of pain 3, 67, 94, 104
 on Krypteia rite 83–84
 on Leonidas 72
 on Lycurgus 72–73, 79, 80, 84, 92, 93
 on Spartan education system 73–74, 102–103
 on Spartan piety 93–94
poinê 43, 44

Popol Vuh 2, 31, 37, 56–64, 158n6
 animals created in 57–58
 animals a failed act of creation in 59, 60, 61, 64
 animal-human binary/hierarchy in 37, 58–60, 64–65
 boundaries/borders in 64–66
 demogonic myth in 62–64
 four-mother fathers in 58, 59, 62, 63, 64
 humans created in 58–59, 60, 62
 Hunahpu/Xbalanque in 61–62
 kinship in 57–59, 64, 65
 mud people/manikins in 58, 59, 61
 origins of myths in 56
 pain (*k'ax*) in 60–64
 sacrifice in 62–63
 speech in 57, 59–60, 63
 terms for pain in 161n38
 translations of 56–57
Poseidon 52
postmodernism 9–10
poststructuralism 1, 2, 7, 10–11, 54
Powell, Anton 70
power 14–15, 26, 38–39, 65, 157n8
 and sexuality 111
 and torture 107, 120
Protestantism 112, 121, 134, 164n10
psychoanalytic theory 7, 11–14
punishment 107, 108
 and Spartan masculinity 74, 77, 78–79

Quirke, Steven 147

race/racism 2, 9, 31, 38, 106, 109, 129–130, 165n4
 see also US white masculinity
rationality/reason 25, 30, 33, 39, 88
Real, the 11, 12, 13, 14
 manufactured 15–16
realism, philosophical 1, 8, 28
Rejali, Darius 4, 110, 163n2
religion 7, 8–9, 121

Rhetorica Christiana (Didacus Valades) 34–36
rites of passage 23, 24, 26–27, 47–48, 91, 118, 157n14, 160n25
    circumcision as 146–148, 152
    see also Apollonian festivals; Artemis-Ortheia, altar of; Krypteia
rituals 2, 3, 24, 25, 26–27, 28, 90
    torture as 109–110, 118–121, 122
Rohingya people 65
Roman period 52, 85, 86, 98, 101, 136
Romanticism 32–33
Römer, Thomas 144
Rosenberg, Jonah 85, 162n4
Roth, Ann Macy 147
Rousseau, Jean-Jacques 37
Ruether, Rosemary Radford 8
Rumsfeld, Donald 109, 114, 116, 165n19

sacrifice 40, 50–51, 52, 54, 56, 59, 90, 94, 97, 101, 121, 161nn28, 29
    ball game (*Popol Vuh*) 62
    circumcision as 13, 140, 142, 143–144, 145, 146, 151, 152, 154
    and divination 83
sadism 4, 108, 110, 129
saints 24, 26, 105
Sanchez, Lt. Gen. Ricardo S. 114, 117–118
Sarajlic, Eldar 133
Sarpedon 48–49, 53, 160n26
Saw, The (Cranach) 27
Sayre, Lewis 126, 132
scarification 26–27, 157n14
Scarry, Elaine 1, 18, 25, 105, 153, 155
science 7, 32, 33–34, 36, 158n10
Scott, Joan W. 16, 21, 154
Scott, Robert 43, 44, 161n34
Sebeok, Thomas A. 1, 6, 7, 10, 18, 20, 22, 90
self 12, 14, 15, 49, 160n27
    and torture 108
semiotics 7, 17–25

    of pain 19–20, 23, 25, 106, 118
    see also icons; indexical sign; symbols
SERE (Survival, Evasion, Resistance, Escape) 111
Sered, Susan 8
Seven Macaw 61, 64
sexuality/sex 29–30, 38, 94, 97, 126, 154
shame 49, 50, 70, 74, 80, 118
sheep 36, 40, 50, 51, 53, 54
Shelemay, Kay Kaufman 17
Shisana, Olive 130
sickles 85, 86–87, 101
Sierra Leone 129
sign-functions 18, 19, 20, 21, 22–23, 28, 157n9
sign-symbols 2, 17, 18, 25, 27, 28, 29, 122, 124–125
signs 18–19, 29, 54
    and body 2
    of the human/non-human animal 23, 31, 37, 39, 42, 65
    as icon/index/symbol 19, 21
    indexical *see* indexical sign
    natural 19–20
    as shifting/in flux 22
Silverman, Kaja 125, 156n3
Silverman, Lisa 17, 24, 109, 163n2, 165n18
Sin City (Miller) 71
Singh, Amrit 111, 115–116, 117, 118, 119, 163nn2, 3, 164n17
slavery 26, 39, 41, 70, 72, 93, 95, 100, 103, 164n18
    see also helots
Snyder, Zack *see* 300 (film/graphic novel, 2007/1998)
social body 133, 149
    and animal–human binary 30, 32, 37, 38, 65
    and pain of animals 51
    penetrated by terrorism 107
social Darwinism 30, 126
social systems/socialization 9
Socrates 76

soul 36, 49, 124, 153, 155
South Africa 129, 130
Sparta 73–76
   governance of 70, 74–75, 76, 79–80, 85, 95
Spartan masculinity 3–4, 67–105, 154
   of Agesilaus 72, 74, 75–76, 95–96
   and Agis 72, 74, 80
   and archeology 68, 84–87
   and austerity 73, 74, 79
   and beautiful death 3, 68, 75, 76–77, 88, 92
   and citizen-soldiers 78
   and clothing/hair/nakedness 68, 78, 81, 88, 91, 92–93, 96, 100
   and *diamastigosis* 69, 84, 98, 99, 101
   and discipline–educational system *see agoge*
   and ephorate/gerousia 75, 85, 88, 89, 92
   failed *see* tremblers
   and festivals of Apollo *see* Apollonian festivals
   and freedom 70, 88–89, 92, 93
   Herodotus on 71, 72, 79
   and Krypteia 69, 83–84, 86, 87, 93, 99–100, 103
   and Leonidas 3–4, 67, 68, 69, 71, 72, 79
   and Lycurgus *see* Lycurgus
   and music 78, 81, 82, 87, 92, 97
   and pain 68, 69, 71–72, 74, 77, 80, 88, 90–91, 94–95, 97, 99, 100, 102, 103
   and piety 89–90, 93–94, 96–97, 101
   Plato on 67, 84, 99
   Plutarch on *see* Plutarch
   and punishment 74, 77, 78–79
   and sexuality 88, 94, 97
   and *300 see 300* (film/graphic novel)
   and treatment of losers in battle 103
   women as upholders of 71, 77
   Xenophon on *see* Xenophon
speciesism 33

speech 2, 38
   authoritative/non-authoritative 41, 47, 111
   in Homeric texts 39, 40–43, 159n16, 160n18
   in *Popol Vuh* 57, 59–60, 63
Spivak, Gayatri 7
stag hunting 39–40, 53, 55, 161n34
stenaxo/stonoeis 44, 46, 160n22
Stevenson, Robert Louis 30
subjectivity 7, 12, 14, 156n7
suffering 17, 43, 44, 45, 136, 160n19, 165n8
symbolic order 11, 12–13, 15
symbols 19, 20, 21–22
   arbitrariness of 22
   and body 23
   and pain 24, 25
   see also sign-symbol
syphilis 127, 133

Taliban *see* torture and war on terror
Tedlock, Dennis 56, 57, 59, 61–62, 63, 64
Tennyson, Alfred 30
terrorism 106–107, 154–155
   and torture *see* torture and the war on terror
textualization 124, 165n1
Thebans 75, 95, 103
theology 8
Thermopylea, Battle of 4, 68, 70, 72, 103
Theron 69, 70, 89, 91–92
Thiessen, Matthew 140, 141
300 (film/graphic novel, 2007/1998) 3–4, 67, 68–72
   agoge in 68–69
   ancient sources for 71, 72
   failed masculinity in 69–70
   freedom in 70, 88–89
   indexical sign of pain in 69, 87, 90–92, 104
   slavery absent in 72, 93, 100
   Spartan women in 71

300 Spartans, The (film, 1962) 72
Tiresias 40
Tiv people 26–27, 157n14
Tohil 62–63
torture 4, 24, 25, 26, 27, 103, 153, 155, 156n2
   and colonialism 129
   and indexical sign of pain *see under* indexical sign of pain
   international conventions on 109, 115
   of Jesus 24, 27, 136, 164n12
   motivations for/types of 108
   as penetration of the body 109, 110–112, 113, 115, 121, 122
   sexual aspects of 108, 110–111, 121
   and truth *see under* truth
torture and war on terror 4, 107–111
   deaths from 117–118, 119, 163n3
   and disentitlement of detainees 115
   and feminization of the other 110–111, 112, 118, 119–120
   and humiliation 106, 110, 111, 116, 117, 118
   and indexical sign of pain 4, 106, 118, 119, 120, 121, 122, 123
   as ineffective/counterproductive 117, 163n2, 164n15
   interrogation methods 116
   legal/political/military discourses on 114–117
   and liminality 109, 115, 118, 119
   and media 109, 114, 117
   and "new paradigm" 115–117, 164n14
   ritualization/rationalization of 109–110, 118–120
   as secret activity 109, 118, 163n5, 164n6
   self-defense rationale for 109, 116
   see also Abu Ghraib
transformation myths 39–40, 61, 158–159n11
tremblers 3, 69–70, 74, 78–79, 80, 87, 89, 91–92, 96, 103, 104, 154

truth
   and body 14, 156n2
   and pain 17, 24, 25, 26, 28, 49, 91, 103, 154, 164–165n19
   and torture 110, 114, 115, 117, 119, 120, 123, 163n2, 164n15, 164–165n18
Tsipporah 142–143, 145, 151, 166n15
Turner, Bryan S. 8
24 (TV series) 114
Tyrtaeus 78

Uexküll, Jakob von 6, 7
Umwelt 6–7, 11, 12, 30–31, 37
unconscious 13, 156n6
United States (US)
   circumcision in 126, 130, 132–133, 149–150
   9/11 attacks in 4, 106–107, 109, 121, 122
   and war on terror *see* torture and war on terror
US white masculinity 106, 110–114, 121–123
   militarized 113–114
   and non-white masculinities 112
   and Protestantism/capitalism 112–113, 121–122, 164n10

van Gennep, Arnold 98, 118, 120, 160n25
Van Howe, Robert 128–129, 132–133
Varley, Lynn 71
Vernant, Jean-Pierre 86, 103
vivisection 25, 26, 131
Vymazalová, Hana 147

war horses 52, 53–54, 56, 161nn30, 31
war on terror 4, 107, 113, 122
   see also torture and war on terror
warfare 45–46, 95, 103, 143–144
   and masculinity 113–114
warrior masculinity 46, 47–50, 56, 66, 143, 154, 159n16, 161n32

see also Israelite warriors; Spartan masculinity
water boarding 119
Weber, Max 112
Weedon, Chris 14, 29, 156*n*3
WHO (World Health Organization) 4, 127, 128, 129, 137, 149, 152
Wisnewski, Jeremy 108, 153, 155
witchcraft 108, 121, 165*n*18
Wolfe, Cary 33
women, and speech 41, 159*n*16
wrath/rage 45–46, 160*n*23

Xbalanque 61, 161*n*37
Xenophon 70, 72, 76–80, 87–88, 95–97, 99
  on Agesilaus 76–77, 95–96, 97
  on *agoge* 77–78, 81, 102–103
  on cheese theft/flagellation ritual 84, 87, 102, 103
  and indexical sign of pain 3, 67, 97, 104
  on Lycurgus 77, 78, 96
  on Spartan religion 89–90
  on Spartan women 77
Xerxes 3, 69, 88, 89
Xibalba 58, 61, 62
Ximénez, Francisco 56, 57
Xmucane 58, 62
xoanon 84, 99, 101, 102
Xpiyaco 58

Yelle, Robert 18, 21, 22, 24
Yoo, John 109, 114, 115–116
Young, Iris Marion 7

Zampieri, Nicola/Zampieri, Cecilia 126
Zeitlin, Froma I. 103
Zeus 38, 39–40, 45, 52, 87, 90, 97, 159*n*11

www.ingramcontent.com/pod-product-compliance
Lightning Source LLC
Chambersburg PA
CBHW062043220426
43662CB00010B/1622